Unlocking Libido

A Woman's Guide to Rediscovering Desire

By
Dr. Katherine M. Reeve

Unlocking Libido

A Woman's Guide to
Rediscovering Desire

Table of Contents

Introduction

Welcome to a journey that promises to illuminate, inspire, and empower you as you navigate the intricate pathways of desire. Low libido is more than just a phase; it's a complex landscape influenced by myriad dimensions of personal, emotional, and physical well-being. For many women, this issue can feel isolating, frustrating, and sometimes insurmountable. But you're not alone, and understanding is the first step towards overcoming it.

This book aims to be your companion, offering insights and practical solutions tailored to your unique experiences and needs. We'll explore the realms of desire, demystifying the factors that influence libido and dispelling myths that have long shadowed women's sexual health. The journey ahead is not just about rekindling sexual desire; it's about embracing a holistic understanding of yourself and the intimate bonds you share with others.

Your story might be different, woven with threads of personal experiences that are unique to your life. Yet, within these pages, you'll find stories, studies, and strategies that resonate with the universal challenges women face regarding libido. Sexual desire is not merely a biological imperative; it's deeply intertwined with the emotional and psychological narratives of our lives. By acknowledging this complexity, you can begin to craft a pathway that leads to a more fulfilling sexual existence.

We'll delve into how societal norms and misconceptions have influenced and, at times, hindered women's sexual lives. Recognising these influences is crucial, but what's equally important is redefining your personal narrative and creating a space where your voice matters. This book encourages you to question the status quo and embrace a sex-positive mindset, championing the importance of open dialogue around sexuality.

Throughout our exploration, you'll find that libido is affected by diverse factors—from the roles of hormones and medication to the impact of emotional well-being and lifestyle choices. Understanding these components is key to navigating the labyrinth of desire. It's not just about identifying the causes but also about empowering yourself with the knowledge to make informed choices that reflect your sexual health and happiness.

Each chapter is crafted to provide a clear, comprehensive understanding of different aspects of libido. We've unpicked the science, dissected psychological factors, and examined the impacts of lifestyle choices on desire. The goal is to build a foundation of knowledge that supports practical application. This journey will equip you with tools to enhance intimacy, whether that means engaging in mindfulness practices, exploring sensuality, or considering alternative therapies.

Importantly, this book also addresses the significant role of relationship dynamics in your sexual health. Communication with your partner is a cornerstone of understanding and improving libido, and this book provides strategies to help you navigate these sometimes delicate conversations. Creating a supportive and open environment with your partner can reignite not only passion but a deeply intimate connection that fuels desire.

Innovation in the realm of sexual health means that there are now more resources available than ever before for those experiencing low libido. From medical interventions to holistic therapies, guided self-discovery, and beyond, we'll explore a range of options that might suit your needs. It's crucial, however, that any action you take aligns with your personal values and comfort levels.

Above all, this journey is about empowerment. Taking charge of your sexual health is a declaration of self-worth and personal agency. It means advocating for yourself in medical, emotional, and relational contexts. The insights and strategies here aim to enhance your confidence and inspire proactive participation in your sexual wellness journey.

Our aim is that by the end of this book, every reader will feel equipped to take actionable steps towards reclaiming and sustaining a vibrant sexual life. With the right support and understanding, the challenges of low libido can transform into a journey of personal growth and fulfillment. As you explore these pages, allow yourself the grace to experiment, reflect, and grow in your unique expression of desire. The path to a satisfying sexual life is not a one-size-fits-all; it's an evolving journey enriched by self-awareness and choice.

Chapter 1:
Understanding Libido

Unearthing the mysteries of female libido can be both enlightening and transformative, especially if you've been experiencing its decline. At its core, libido is a complex interplay of biological signals, emotional states, and intimate connections. Each woman experiences it uniquely, shaped by individual desires and circumstances. Understanding this dynamic energy involves embracing the science behind it without losing sight of the human element. While science offers insights into neurotransmitters and hormonal influences, it's essential to acknowledge the myriad factors that contribute to how desire manifests. These factors can range from psychological aspects such as stress and self-perception to lifestyle influences like diet and daily routines. By delving into these intricacies, you'll not only gain clarity on the multifaceted nature of libido but also recognise the empowerment that comes from being in tune with your desires. This knowledge is your first step towards reclaiming a fulfilling and passionate life, where intimacy is not just physical, but also an enriching connection with yourself and your partner.

The Science Behind Female Desire

The intricacies of female desire are a tapestry woven from various threads, each contributing to the complex pattern of libido. At its core, desire is influenced by a sophisticated interplay of biological, psychological, and socio-cultural factors. To begin unravelling this complexity, we must dive into the science that forms desire's foundation, acknowledging the nuances and subtleties that make female libido unique.

From a biological standpoint, hormones play a pivotal role in regulating sexual desire. Oestrogen and testosterone, though often discussed in contexts involving puberty or menopause, have significant impacts on libido throughout a woman's life. Oestrogen is known for maintaining vaginal health and lubrication, which naturally contributes to sexual comfort and, therefore, desire. Testosterone, albeit present in lower levels than in men, is crucial for fuelling sexual arousal and libido. Hormonal fluctuations during the menstrual cycle can lead to varying levels of desire, with some women experiencing increased libido at specific times, such as mid-cycle around ovulation.

Beyond hormones, the brain serves as an essential command centre where sexual desire originates. The limbic system, particularly the hypothalamus, is instrumental in processing sexual stimuli and triggering feelings of desire. Neurotransmitters, such as dopamine and serotonin, further influence these feelings. Dopamine is associated with pleasure and reward, often linked with the anticipation of sexual experiences, while serotonin can both suppress and enhance desire depending on its levels and balance with other chemicals in the brain.

The psychological dimensions of desire are equally significant. Mental health states, including stress, anxiety, and depression, can substantially impact a woman's libido. Stress, for instance, activates the body's fight-or-flight response, releasing cortisol, which can inhibit sexual desire and dampen arousal. Furthermore, women who perceive themselves as highly stressed may find it challenging to switch gears from the mental juggling of daily tasks to a mindful, present state conducive to intimacy.

Differentiating between spontaneous and responsive desire also provides insight into the variability of female libido. Spontaneous desire is immediate and arises without external stimuli, akin to a reflexive urge. In contrast, responsive desire develops more gradually and in response to an experience or interaction, suggesting that context and emotion significantly influence female sexual interest.

Socio-cultural influences on desire shouldn't be underestimated. Society's narratives and expectations regarding female sexuality can shape how women perceive their own desires. Throughout history, women's sexual desire has been confined by societal norms, leading to stigmatization or misinterpretation. The cultural script around 'normal' libido can create unnecessary pressure, sometimes affecting a woman's genuine understanding of her own desires and needs.

Furthermore, personal upbringing and past experiences contribute to an individual's sexual identity and desire. Early exposure to attitudes about sex and relationships, either through family teaching or sociocultural narratives, can surface later in life, impacting libido. The process from which women often have to disentangle these inherited notions and construct their unique sexual self is complex but empowering.

Adding another layer, recent studies suggest that access to satisfying and enriching relationships also significantly enhances desire. Emotional intimacy fosters a sense of security and trust, which can naturally elevate libido. The connection between emotional and physical intimacy illustrates that desire is often cultivated in nurturing spaces where emotional needs are met.

In contrast, negative experiences like trauma or unhealthy relationships can disrupt the flow of desire. Understanding the ramifications of such experiences is vital for healing and regaining a healthy perspective on sexuality. It's crucial for women to feel safe and supported in any relationship dynamic to embrace their sexual identity fully.

Lifestyle factors, while often overlooked, are instrumental in influencing libido. Exercise and nutrition not only boost physical health but also enhance mental clarity and mood, which can directly impact sexual desire. Regular physical activity increases endorphins and improves circulation, fostering better sexual functioning and interest. A balanced diet can help in maintaining optimal hormonal levels, contributing to a well-regulated libido.

Understanding the science behind female desire provides an invaluable framework for women seeking to comprehend their sexual selves. It's a scientific dialogue, one that respects individual variability and encourages personal exploration. Each woman is unique, and recognising personal patterns and contexts, while also being informed by science, can lead to a more intentional and empowered approach to sexual health and satisfaction.

Ultimately, education about the science of desire can help demystify the process, break down stigma, and create room for genuine self-expression and satisfaction. Equipping oneself with this knowledge is a step towards reclaiming control over one's sexual narrative, paving the way for a more fulfilling and harmonious intimate life.

Factors Affecting Libido

Libido can be a mysterious aspect of our lives. It's a personal journey—one shaped by a myriad of factors. Just as a symphony is influenced by each instrumental note, a woman's desire is moulded by an intricate interplay of elements. Let's delve into these factors, acknowledging that each woman's experience is unique, an orchestration of both physiological and psychological components.

First and foremost, the delicate balance of hormones plays a pivotal role. The ebb and flow of oestrogen and testosterone can significantly shape a woman's sexual desire. These hormones influence the physical mechanisms of arousal and readiness, yet they also affect mood and energy levels. It's this fascinating intersection between body and mind that underscores the need for holistic awareness when addressing libido issues. During certain life phases like menopause or postpartum, these hormonal shifts are even more pronounced, sometimes leading to a noticeable dip in desire.

Beyond the biological, emotional well-being acts as a cornerstone of sexual desire. Stress and overwhelming responsibilities might burden you, leading to a diminished interest in intimacy. The pressures of modern life, with its deadlines and demands, can steal away the mental space required for passion to flourish. Here, mindfulness and stress reduction techniques come into play, fostering a more serene mental landscape where desire can thrive.

Relationship dynamics are equally influential. The emotional bond—built on trust, communication, and intimacy—directly affects a woman's libido. Misunderstandings or unresolved conflicts with a partner can act like a formidable block in the pathway of sexual desire. It's imperative to nurture open conversations, which in turn promote a deeper connection and rekindle that spark of interest in one another.

Physical health can't be overlooked in this equation. Think of energy levels and how they affect your overall sense of well-being. Engaging in regular exercise not only boosts physical vitality but also releases endorphins—the body's natural mood lifters. These enhance a woman's sense of attractiveness and desirability, often translating into a heightened libido.

Not to be underestimated, lifestyle choices like nutrition can also impact sexual desire. A balanced diet rich in essential nutrients supports overall health, including hormonal health, which in turn influences libido. For instance, essential fatty acids found in foods like avocados and nuts can boost the body's ability to naturally regulate sexual hormones. Conversely, poor nutrition and habits like excessive alcohol or caffeine intake might impair sexual responsiveness and interest.

Sleep, though frequently underrated, is a key player in maintaining sexual drive. Adequate rest supports optimal hormone function and emotional balance. Imagine a vicious cycle where lack of sleep leads to stress and irritability, consequently reducing the appetite for intimacy. Attending to sleep hygiene can bring about significant improvements in sexual desire.

Psychological factors, such as past traumas or present anxieties, are also at the heart of libido. They often linger quietly but can profoundly affect one's willingness to engage in intimate encounters. Addressing these psychological wounds with compassion, perhaps through therapy, can unlock potential for restored desire and fulfilment.

Societal and cultural narratives also weave through the fabric of libido, sometimes in subtle ways. Society often imposes expectations about what is deemed 'normal' in terms of sexual desires, timelines, and performances. The pressure to conform to these norms can inhibit genuine expressions of desire, creating a disconnect between what one feels and what one thinks they should feel.

Medication can't be ignored in this conversation. Many commonly prescribed medications, including antidepressants and anti-hypertensives, list reduced libido as a side effect. It's crucial to discuss these effects openly with healthcare professionals to find possible alternatives or manage these unwanted consequences effectively.

In the world of connectivity and digital presence, social media can influence libido too. Constant engagement in virtual spaces might detract from real-world connections. Furthermore, the portrayal of idealised relationships and bodies online can create dissatisfaction and performance anxiety, affecting real-life sexual desire.

Lastly, environmental factors also play their part. Everything from the lighting of a bedroom to the presence of technology in intimate spaces can alter a woman's readiness for intimacy. A supportive environment that maximises comfort and warmth can create an inviting atmosphere for desire to flourish.

Unravelling the factors affecting libido is much like piecing together a puzzle. It requires curiosity, patience, and an open heart. Understanding these varied influences empowers women to navigate their paths, paving the way towards a fulfilling and vibrant sexual life.

Chapter 2:
Exploring the Myths

As we delve into the realm of myths surrounding female libido, it's crucial to unravel the stories that have been told and retold, often leading to misunderstandings and unnecessary guilt. The myth that a woman's desire is simple and predictable is not only outdated but also fundamentally flawed. Our desires are as diverse and dynamic as we are, shaped by a complex interplay of personal, cultural, and societal factors. Breaking free from these myths allows us to view low libido not as a flaw, but as a natural variation deserving of empathy and understanding. Disentangling these misconceptions offers a liberating perspective, one that recognizes the unique and individualized nature of every woman's sexual desire. It's this fresh lens that empowers you to navigate your journey with greater clarity and confidence, redefining what desire means on your terms. Together, let's embrace the truth that our sexual selves are multifaceted, ever-evolving, and deserving of genuine curiosity and care.

Debunking Common Misconceptions

When it comes to female libido, myths and misconceptions abound. They've woven themselves into the very fabric of our understanding, often going unchallenged and leaving us with false narratives that only deepen the confusion and frustration many women feel. Let's shine a light on these misconceptions and explore the truths behind them, helping you to reclaim your desire and dispel the shadows of misinformation.

One prevalent myth is that libido is a switch that's either "on" or "off." This simplistic view overlooks the complexity and fluidity of female sexual desire. Libido isn't a static entity but rather a spectrum of feelings that can fluctuate throughout your life for numerous reasons. Stress, medications, hormonal changes, and relationship dynamics are just a few factors that can influence your sexual desire. Understanding that it's natural for libido to ebb and flow allows for a more compassionate and realistic approach to dealing with changes in desire.

Another common misconception is the idea that women should always have an innate desire for sex. Societal influences can often portray male desire as constant and overwhelming, leading to a belief that if women don't feel the same way, there's something inherently wrong with them. This comparison is not only inaccurate but also detrimental. Female sexuality is fundamentally responsive rather than spontaneous, a concept expertly defined by researchers. Desire can be prompted by intimacy and emotional connection, often overlapping with other aspects of a woman's life, rather than being an ever-present urge.

It's also frequently believed that low libido is a symptom that will eventually fix itself. However, without addressing the underlying causes, it may linger and even intensify. This passive approach often delays valuable opportunities for healing and rediscovery. By recognising when your desire is waning, you create space for proactive change, whether through counselling, lifestyle adjustments, or improved communication with your partner.

A particularly damaging misconception is that a woman's libido is inherently less important than her partner's. This skewed perspective can foster feelings of inadequacy and resentment, adversely affecting both intimacy and self-worth. Every individual's sexual health is crucial, and when both partners prioritise open dialogue and mutual fulfilment, relationships tend to flourish. Understanding your needs and voicing them is not just an act of bravery; it's a cornerstone of a healthy sexual life.

Another myth suggests that aging inevitably leads to an uninterested sex life. While hormonal shifts during menopause can affect desire, this doesn't mean passion can't be maintained or even reignited. In fact, many women find that with the freedom from contraception worries and children's demands, they can explore new dimensions of their sexuality with more confidence and enthusiasm. Realigning expectations and embracing new approaches can lead to a deeply rewarding sexual experience at any age.

There's also a misconception that libido is primarily driven by physical attraction and nothing more. In reality, emotional connection, mental stimulation, and body confidence play significant roles in how desire manifests. While visual attraction can certainly be a part of the equation, it is by no means the entirety of it. Cultivating a deeper emotional bond, exploring sensuality, and enhancing body awareness contribute to desire in profound ways.

We also find the age-old myth that sexual desire should naturally be as strong throughout long-term relationships as it was during the initial stages. The fiery passion of early romance often evolves into a more nuanced and profound connection. It's a normal and healthy transition. Recognising this evolution and working to understand and appreciate your current place in that journey can bring a new sense of gratitude and intention to your sexual relationship.

Lastly, there is a belief that low libido should only be addressed through medical or therapeutic interventions. While these can be incredibly effective, they are not the sole avenues for revitalising desire. Embracing holistic approaches to wellness, such as mindfulness, yoga, and attending to nutritional needs, can enhance libido by boosting overall wellbeing. A balanced approach that incorporates physical, emotional, and psychological facets can provide the most effective pathway to renewed desire.

By debunking these myths, we not only remove the stigma surrounding low libido but also pave the way for genuine understanding and empowerment. With knowledge in hand, you can choose the steps that resonate with your unique experience. Embrace the fluidity of your sexual journey, knowing that it doesn't need to conform to societal narratives or expectations. Each myth unraveled is a step toward dispelling doubt and embracing a fulfilling and dynamic sexual life.

Societal Influences on Female Libido

Throughout history, societal expectations have played a significant role in shaping the narrative surrounding female libido. These influences are so deeply embedded in culture that they often dictate how women perceive their own desires and sexual appetites. It's not just about what society says overtly; it's also about the subtle cues and norms that pervade our everyday lives. From the media we consume to the conversations we overhear, the narrative around female desire has been shaped by external factors, often leaving women feeling disconnected from their true selves.

At the heart of the issue lies a historical context where male sexuality was often openly discussed and accepted, while female sexuality was shrouded in mystery, modesty, or even shame. The traditional patriarchal view that prioritises male pleasure over female experiences has left its mark, creating a myth that women's libido is less potent or important. This results in women internalising unrealistic expectations about what a 'normal' libido should look like, often leading to feelings of inadequacy or confusion when their experiences don't align with these societal presumptions.

The media paints a picture that women's sexual desire should resemble an endless honeymoon phase or that it exists purely for male enjoyment. This portrayal isn't just misleading; it actively contributes to the myth that a woman's libido is a simple, unchanging facet of her nature. In reality, female libido is as unique and dynamic as the women themselves, influenced by a myriad of factors that cannot be boiled down to a one-size-fits-all template. Yet, the pervasive depiction of female sexuality in movies, television, and advertisements insists otherwise, often leading women to doubt the legitimacy of their own sexual experiences.

Peer pressure and societal norms further complicate the landscape. In many communities, discussing one's sexual needs or desires is still considered taboo, perpetuating the idea that such conversations are inappropriate for women. This silence only deepens the mystery and confusion around female libido, making women less likely to seek help or discuss their concerns. When female sexual desires are relegated to the shadows, it becomes almost impossible for women to embrace their sexuality openly and without fear. This cultural silence thus becomes another barrier for women trying to understand and improve their libido.

Education, or rather the lack of comprehensive sexual education, compounds the problem. Many women receive inadequate information about their own bodies, sexual anatomy, and the complexities of desire, leading to misunderstandings about what is 'normal.' Schools often focus on reproductive health without delving into concepts of pleasure or desire. When society fails to educate women about their own bodies, it leaves them vulnerable to internalising harmful stereotypes and struggling with unmet sexual expectations.

Religious and cultural influences also play significant roles in moulding perceptions of female libido. In some settings, women are taught from an early age that expressing or even acknowledging sexual desire is sinful or shameful. These teachings can create a rift between a woman's natural inclinations and societal expectations, leading to guilt and anxiety around sexual experiences. Such influences can deeply impact a woman's self-perception, making it harder for her to accept desire as a healthy and normal aspect of being human.

Despite these challenges, it's crucial to recognise that societal norms are not fixed. They evolve over time, shaped by the ever-changing voices and actions of individuals and communities. Women today are redefining sexuality on their own terms, challenging stereotypes, and debunking myths. The growing movement towards sexual empowerment sees women of all ages, backgrounds, and orientations advocating for their right to experience desire unencumbered by outdated societal constructs.

Open conversations and a growing body of literature focused on female sexuality are helping to lift the veil, offering positive narratives that celebrate rather than suppress sexual desire. As society becomes more inclusive and accepting of diverse experiences, women are finding strength in sharing their stories, often discovering commonalities in what once felt like isolated struggles. This shift is not just vital for individual women, but for society as a whole, helping to foster environments where open dialogue and acceptance can thrive.

Recognising the societal influences on female libido is the first step towards empowering women to forge their paths. By understanding how external pressures shape perceptions and acknowledging their impact, women can begin to separate myth from reality. In doing so, they lay the groundwork for a more authentic and fulfilling exploration of their desires. It's about reclaiming ownership of one's body and experiences, and most importantly, redefining what it means to desire in a way that is bold, beautiful, and entirely one's own.

Ultimately, the journey to understanding and embracing female libido is a personal one. It's about recognising and challenging the societal influences that have informed this journey and moving toward a future where female desire is celebrated rather than criticised. As more women embrace this empowerment movement, they contribute to shifting the narrative, ensuring that future generations will grow up in a world that recognises and honours the full spectrum of female sexual desire.

Chapter 3:
Identifying Causes of Low Libido

As we delve into the multifaceted nature of low libido, it's crucial to recognise that its causes are as diverse as they are interconnected. Psychological factors, such as underlying stress or past traumas, can cast long shadows on one's desire, intertwining with physiological contributors like hormonal imbalances or medical conditions. Meanwhile, lifestyle choices, encompassing everything from sleep patterns to dietary habits, can subtly erode sexual desire over time. Each of these elements doesn't exist in a vacuum but forms a complex tapestry that can leave many women feeling disconnected from their sexual selves. By identifying and understanding these causes, you empower yourself to take the first steps toward rediscovering and rekindling your innate desire, transforming what may feel like a struggle into a journey of personal growth and self-discovery.

Psychological Factors in Low Libido

Low libido in women can often be intricately linked to psychological factors, forming a delicate tapestry of emotions and experiences. It's not unusual for women to find that their mental and emotional states deeply affect their levels of sexual desire. This connection between mind and libido can become particularly poignant during periods of psychological distress or emotional upheaval. Indeed, the complexities of the psyche hold significant sway over the sexual aspects of our lives, sometimes in ways that are not immediately apparent.

A key psychological factor influencing libido is stress. Whether it stems from work, family responsibilities, or financial concerns, stress can pervade every aspect of life, leading to a diminished interest in sex. The mind, preoccupied with anxiety and tension, often leaves little room for the spontaneity and relaxation that sexual desire requires. Stress activates the body's fight-or-flight response, flooding the system with hormones like cortisol, which can dampen libido over time. Creating spaces for relaxation and mindfulness can help mitigate these effects, paving the way for a resurgence in desire.

Self-esteem and body image issues also weigh heavily on psychological well-being and, consequently, libido. In a world where societal standards of beauty are relentlessly promoted, many women struggle with self-doubt about their bodies, undermining their confidence during intimate moments. This negative self-perception can greatly impact one's ability to enjoy and pursue sexual intimacy. Rediscovering self-confidence often involves a compassionate reevaluation of one's body and self-worth, supported by reinforcing positive self-talk and surrounding oneself with affirming narratives.

Another influential psychological factor is past trauma. Women who've experienced sexual or emotional trauma may encounter significant barriers to libido. These experiences can cause emotional scarring, manifesting as aversion or anxiety related to sexual activities. Healing from such trauma is a deeply personal journey that may require professional support, such as therapy, and the establishment of a safe and supportive environment to rebuild trust in oneself and others. Addressing these traumas with sensitivity and patience can lead to profound liberation and rekindled desire.

Furthermore, relational dynamics profoundly affect psychological states and, by extension, libido. The emotional climate within a relationship can either nurture or hinder sexual desire. Tensions and unresolved conflicts with a partner can erode the emotional intimacy necessary for a healthy sex life. Open communication, empathy, and mutual support form the bedrock of emotional and sexual connection, laying the groundwork for a vibrant sexual relationship. Couples can benefit from taking time to reconnect and rebuild trust, significantly revitalising their shared intimacy.

Additionally, the influence of societal expectations on women's sexual roles cannot be overlooked. Societal norms often dictate what is "acceptable" when it comes to female desire, leading to feelings of shame or guilt about sexual wants and needs. These expectations can be internalised, resulting in a decreased libido. Challenging and redefining these norms on a personal level involves embracing one's sexual identity with pride and recognising the legitimacy of one's desires without shame.

Anxiety and depression are also significant psychological factors that can lead to low libido. The symptoms of these mental health conditions—such as persistent sadness, fatigue, and lack of interest—can drastically reduce sexual desire. Treatment often involves addressing the underlying anxiety or depression with the help of mental health professionals, and may include therapy, medication, or lifestyle adjustments. As mental well-being improves, libido often sees an uptick as emotional resilience and joie de vivre begin to return.

Moreover, emotional burnout—which can arise from overcommitment and lack of self-care—impacts both mental health and libido. Women often find themselves juggling multiple roles, leading to exhaustion not only physically but emotionally and mentally. When burnout takes hold, the instinct to conserve energy for essential activities often overtakes the desire for sexual intimacy. Recognising the signs of burnout and implementing strategies for self-care, such as setting boundaries and creating time for rest, are essential steps toward recovery.

Beyond individual factors, it's crucial to consider how a holistic understanding of these psychological elements can be woven into a broader strategy to enhance libido. This understanding should be rooted in a compassionate view of oneself, recognising that psychological well-being is integral to sexual health. By acknowledging and addressing these psychological underpinnings, women can empower themselves to overcome the hurdles of low libido and move toward a more satisfying and enriched sexual life.

In conclusion, psychological factors play a pivotal role in shaping libido, capable of both stifling and reigniting desire. By exploring and addressing these intricate influences, women can take pivotal steps toward reclaiming their sexuality. Armed with greater awareness and understanding, it's entirely possible to forge a path toward a more passionate and fulfilling sexual existence—one that honours both the complexity of the mind and the rich tapestry of desire.

Physiological Factors in Low Libido

Understanding the physiological aspects that may contribute to low libido is essential in the journey to revitalise sexual desire. The body isn't merely a vehicle through which we experience the world; it's an integral part of our sexual identity. Various physiological elements can influence libido, and recognising these can provide valuable insights and solutions.

Hormonal imbalances are among the most significant physiological factors affecting libido. Hormones like oestrogen, progesterone, and testosterone play vital roles in sexual desire. For instance, as women approach menopause, a natural decline in oestrogen can lead to changes in libido. It's not just about the feeling of desire but also physical symptoms, such as vaginal dryness, that can make intimacy less appealing. Understanding these changes and considering hormone replacement therapy, after consulting with a healthcare provider, might offer relief and rejuvenation.

Furthermore, thyroid function is another critical component influencing libido. Hypothyroidism, characterised by a sluggish thyroid, can lead to low energy levels, weight gain, and mood fluctuations, all of which can collectively dampen sexual desire. Identifying thyroid issues through medical consultation and appropriate treatment can help restore balance, both physically and emotionally.

The role of neurological conditions can't be ignored when discussing physiological influences on libido. Disorders like multiple sclerosis or Parkinson's disease impact the nervous system, which in turn affects sexual function and desire. These conditions can lead to physical discomfort or reduced sensitivity, making sexual experiences less pleasurable. Consulting a neurologist or seeking specialised therapy can significantly aid in managing symptoms and finding adaptive techniques to enhance intimacy.

Physical health conditions, such as diabetes or hypertension, also have far-reaching implications for libido. Diabetes, in particular, can cause nerve damage and impact blood flow, leading to sexual dysfunction. Similarly, some medications used to control high blood pressure may contribute to decreased libido. Addressing these health issues with a medical professional can improve not only overall well-being but also revive sexual interest.

Chronic pain conditions, including arthritis or fibromyalgia, can alter the body's capacity for sexual desire by causing uncomfortable sensations during sexual activity. The persistent nature of pain can be exhausting, mentally and physically, deterring intimate encounters. Discovering pain management strategies, including medical and holistic approaches, can facilitate a more fulfilling sexual life.

It is crucial to consider contraception methods as well. Certain birth control pills can have side effects that influence libido due to alterations in hormone levels. Discussing alternative options with a healthcare provider may help in identifying the most suitable contraceptive that doesn't compromise sexual desire.

Moreover, breastfeeding mothers often experience shifts in libido due to hormonal changes and the physical demands of childcare. The hormone prolactin, which supports milk production, naturally reduces sexual desire. Understanding that this phase is temporary can relieve pressure and allow a more patient approach to rekindling intimacy over time.

Lastly, it's imperative to highlight the impact of surgical interventions. Procedures such as hysterectomy or mastectomy can have profound emotional and physical repercussions on a woman's sense of sexuality and desirability. Recovery is both a physical and emotional journey, and seeking support from mental health professionals, along with physical therapy, can be invaluable in rediscovering one's sexual identity.

Awareness of these physiological factors empowers women to engage in informed conversations with healthcare providers. Armed with this knowledge, you can explore comprehensive strategies tailored to individual needs. After all, understanding the body isn't about accepting limitations but rather about seeking possibilities to thrive and embrace a satisfying, passionate life.

Lifestyle Impacts on Libido

Our daily routines and choices significantly shape our sexual desire, often in ways we might not immediately recognise. From the hustle of our work schedules to the subtleties of our sleep patterns, every facet of our lifestyle can play a role in either nurturing or diminishing libido.

Understanding these impacts is crucial to navigating and overcoming low libido challenges.

First, consider the impact of stress. Modern life can be relentless with its demands and responsibilities, and it's often stress that takes the front seat. The body's response to stress involves the release of cortisol, a hormone that can suppress sexual desire. Chronic stress can lead to a cycle where anxiety and a feeling of being overwhelmed erode any remnants of libido. To combat this, integrative approaches such as yoga, meditation, or breathing exercises can be vital. These practices not only improve mental well-being but also support a more positive and relaxed state that is conducive to desire.

Sleep, often an underrated factor, plays an essential role in sexual health. Poor quality sleep or insufficient rest can lead to irritability, fatigue, and even depression—all of which are barriers to sexual interest. Ensuring a regular sleep schedule and creating a calming bedtime routine, free from digital distractions, can rejuvenate energy levels and positively impact libido. Consistent restful nights can lead to improved mood, enhanced energy, and a more profound sense of wellbeing, all of which underpin a healthy sexual appetite.

Diet is another critical aspect often overlooked. A balanced diet provides the body with all the necessary nutrients to function optimally, including in the realm of sexual health. Foods rich in zinc, omega-3 fatty acids, and antioxidants support hormone production and circulation, key components of libido. Conversely, diets high in processed foods, sugars, and unhealthy fats can impede sexual function. It might be useful to incorporate nutrient-dense foods, such as nuts, seeds, lean proteins, and leafy greens, to enhance overall vitality, thereby supporting a vibrant sexual desire.

Exercise, too, has multifaceted benefits for sexual desire. Physical activity boosts endorphin levels, increases blood flow, and promotes better self-perception, all of which can contribute to a heightened libido. Regular exercise can help in alleviating symptoms of stress, depression, and anxiety by releasing "feel-good" hormones. Furthermore, exercise enhances physical confidence, which translates into greater sexual confidence and willingness to engage in intimate encounters.

Social connections, or the lack thereof, can also impact desire. Human beings are inherently social creatures, and meaningful interactions contribute to mental health and, by extension, sexual health. Connection with others nurtures our emotional needs, and feeling supported can lead to a stronger sense of self-worth and body confidence, potentially reigniting a waning libido.

Moreover, lifestyle habits such as alcohol and substance use can affect libido. While a glass of wine might help you relax on occasion, excessive consumption can impair sexual function. Alcohol acts as a depressant and can disrupt the delicate balance of hormones necessary for a healthy libido. Reducing or moderating intake might result in noticeable improvements in sexual desire.

It's important to mention the role of digital exposure. The ubiquitous presence of smartphones and screens often results in the neglect of real-world interactions. Engaging more with the physical environment rather than the virtual one can improve mental focus and emotional readiness for intimacy. Establishing tech-free zones or times within your day for personal connection can help nurture sexual desire.

In summary, our lifestyle choices play an intricate role in either enhancing or diminishing sexual desire. By addressing areas like stress management, sleep quality, diet, exercise, and social interactions, women can positively influence their libido. While it may seem overwhelming to reconsider these habits, taking small, consistent steps can lead to significant changes over time. Remember, revamping your lifestyle in favour of better sexual health is not solely about making changes for better sex; it's about enhancing your quality of life and overall well-being. By taking proactive steps to modify these everyday factors, you can pave the way to rediscovering and rekindling your sexual desire, ultimately leading to a more fulfilling, empowered, and intimate life.

Chapter 4:
Emotional and Psychological
Well-being

Understanding and nurturing your emotional and psychological well-being is crucial in the journey to rekindle your libido. It's easy to overlook how deeply intertwined our emotional states are with our sexual desire. Feelings of stress, anxiety, and even depression can create barriers, making it difficult for desire to flourish. Imagine trying to light a fire when rain keeps pouring down; emotional distress can have a similar dampening effect on your libido. Recognising these challenges as part of a larger picture allows you to address them with compassion and intention. You have the power to transform how you feel emotionally, and this change can pave the way for renewed desire. Embrace the opportunity to listen to what your mind and body are telling you, and take steps to foster a balanced and nurturing environment for your psyche. As you cultivate emotional resilience, you'll find a newfound sense of empowerment, opening the door to a more fulfilling and intimate connection with yourself and your partner.

How Stress Affects Desire

It's truly fascinating how stress can weave itself into the tapestry of our lives, affecting nearly every aspect, including our sexual desire. This thread of tension, inseparable from daily living, often goes unnoticed until it tightens its grip. In many ways, stress acts like an invisible barrier between you and your natural desires. Understanding this connection more deeply requires us to untangle the complex relationship between stress and libido.

First, let's consider the physiological changes that occur under stress. When faced with a stressful situation, your body gets flooded with cortisol, the primary stress hormone. It's your body's natural response designed to handle short-term dangers. Unfortunately, when stress becomes chronic, cortisol levels can soar persistently, leading to a decrease in sexual desire. This diversion of energy prioritises survival rather than reproduction. The body becomes focused on facing threats rather than nurturing intimacy.

Beyond the biochemical reactions, stress influences libido through mental and emotional pathways. Imagine trying to feel intimate when your mind is preoccupied with a never-ending to-do list or looming deadlines. Such mental distractions make it incredibly difficult to be present and engage in the moment, which is essential for experiencing desire and pleasure.

It's not just the immediate stress that takes a toll. Long-term exposure can lead to anxiety and depressive symptoms, further distancing you from your desires. As the world turns increasingly fast-paced, the stressors pile up, leaving little room for relaxation and enjoyment. Emotional bandwidth becomes occupied with managing tensions rather than indulging in life's pleasures. This state of constant vigilance contributes to a cycle where intimacy is pushed to the back burner.

The emotional burden of stress can create tension in personal relationships, exacerbating the issue. When you're stressed, your patience may fray, communication can break down, and misunderstandings arise more frequently. It's a setup for frustration and conflict rather than connection and desire. Knowing this, it's imperative to address stress not only as a personal issue but also as one that affects the dynamics of your relationship.

There's an empowering realisation in understanding the impact of stress: you can take steps to manage it. Engaging in activities that promote relaxation can significantly enhance your emotional and psychological well-being. Techniques such as mindfulness, deep breathing, and regular physical exercise might already sound familiar because they've been proven through research to lower stress levels. When stress is managed, libido often finds its way back to being a priority.

Consider also the significance of self-care. In a world where productivity is highly valued, taking time for oneself can feel indulgent. But it's crucial for replenishing your emotional reserves. Whether it's soaking in a warm bath, engaging in hobbies, or simply ensuring you get enough rest, these nurturing actions are foundational to reducing stress and reviving desire. It's about giving yourself permission to slow down and nurture your own needs.

Moreover, evaluating the sources of stress in your life with a critical eye can be transformative. Some stressors may be external, like work demands, while others could be internal, like personal expectations and self-criticism. By identifying these and addressing them either through setting healthy boundaries or adjusting your expectations, you can carve out space for more positive experiences and intimacy.

Another powerful tool is open communication with your partner. Sharing feelings of stress and its impacts can foster understanding and support. When your partner is aware of what you're going through, they can provide the support and patience needed to navigate these challenges together. It can also open the door to find new ways of connecting that weren't previously considered.

Stress is a normal part of life, but its impact on sexual desire doesn't have to be accepted as an unchangeable reality. By taking proactive steps to manage stress and its effects, you can create an environment where desire thrives. Remember that rekindling this aspect of your life is a journey, not a destination. It involves patience, exploration, and the willingness to make adjustments as needed.

The path toward a fulfilling sexual life amid stress is about acknowledging the influence it has and choosing to take action. It's a dance between managing what life throws at you and setting the stage for intimacy to flourish. Through intentional efforts and emotional honesty, you're moving towards a fulfilling connection with your own desires and with your partner.

Addressing Anxiety and Depression

Understanding the complex interplay between anxiety, depression, and libido is pivotal in tackling the challenges of low sexual desire. Emotional and psychological well-being profoundly impact sexual health, and for many women, these factors hold the key to understanding fluctuations in libido. Anxiety and depression can create a vicious cycle, where decreased libido heightens stress and emotional disturbances, leading to further deterioration in desire.

Anxiety often manifests in the incessant buzzing of worries, casting a shadow over every aspect of life, including sexual intimacy. This heightened state of alertness—constantly fearing the worst or feeling pressured by perfection—can obstruct relaxation, a key component needed for sexual arousal and enjoyment. The mind races, and it becomes nearly impossible to immerse oneself in the moment or feel connected to one's partner. This disconnect can lead to frustration, further escalating feelings of anxiety, and creating a self-perpetuating loop of stress.

Depression, on the other hand, tends to dull emotions and energy levels, making the pursuit of sexual connection feel arduous at best. The common symptoms of depression include fatigue, lack of interest in previously enjoyed activities, and a general sense of hopelessness—all of which can steal away the joy and pleasure that come with sexual intimacy. As life seems to lose its colour and vibrancy, sexual desire can wane, resulting in a feeling of isolation even within intimate partnerships.

However, acknowledging and addressing these mental health challenges can open the door to reclaiming one's libido. It's important to recognise that there is no shame in experiencing anxiety or depression, nor in seeking help to manage these conditions. Opening up about these feelings, whether to a trusted friend, partner, or mental health professional, can relieve the burden of carrying these emotions alone. This can also initiate a path to healing and emotional recovery, which can in turn improve sexual well-being.

Therapeutic approaches, such as cognitive-behavioural therapy (CBT), have been shown to effectively reduce symptoms of anxiety and depression. CBT focuses on identifying and challenging unhealthy thought patterns and beliefs that contribute to emotional distress. For women experiencing low libido linked to these mental health issues, CBT can help shift their internal narrative, creating room for self-compassion and acceptance. Understanding and reworking these thought patterns can also enhance communication with partners, fostering an environment of support and intimacy.

Mindfulness practices can be particularly beneficial in managing anxiety and depression. These practices involve cultivating an awareness of the present moment through techniques such as meditation, deep breathing, and body scanning. By anchoring oneself in the present, mindfulness can help interrupt the cycle of anxious or depressive thoughts, allowing for a more conscious and intentional engagement with oneself and one's partner. When the mind is calmer and more centred, it becomes easier to attune to desires and sensations, potentially reigniting sparks of libido.

While navigating anxiety and depression, it's crucial to maintain an open dialogue with one's partner. Transparency about emotional struggles can lead to compassionate understanding and patience within the relationship. By sharing one's experiences and needs, partners can work collaboratively to find solutions and adapt their intimacy to reflect the current reality. This mutual effort can strengthen the relationship bond, reinforcing a sense of unity and shared resilience.

Self-care also plays a critical role in managing anxiety and depression. Establishing a routine that nurtures both body and mind—including regular physical activity, sufficient rest, and balanced nutrition—can create a stable foundation for emotional well-being. These practices not only improve mood but also enhance physical health, directly supporting sexual desire by boosting energy levels and increasing the resilience needed to face emotional challenges.

For some women, medication may be a necessary component of treating anxiety or depression. It's important to have open conversations with healthcare providers about the effects these medications might have on libido. Some antidepressants, for instance, are known to affect sexual desire negatively, and adjustments to treatment plans might be needed. Prioritising mental health is paramount, but it's also essential to explore options that best align with an individual's overall well-being and sexual health goals.

Ultimately, addressing anxiety and depression is a journey of reclaiming one's life and sexuality. By understanding the connection between emotional health and libido, women can embark on a transformative process of healing. This path involves courageously facing emotional difficulties, seeking support when needed, and maintaining openness and vulnerability with oneself and others.

Through resilience and dedication to emotional well-being, it is possible to rediscover desire in a renewed, empowering light.

This journey is unique to every individual, requiring personalized strategies and approaches. Yet, the rewards of engaging with and overcoming these emotional challenges can lead to a revitalised sense of self and a deeply fulfilling intimate connection. Embracing this process not only empowers women to reignite their passions but also fosters a holistic approach to living that honours both mental health and sexual vitality.

Chapter 5:
Physical Health and Libido

The intricate dance between physical health and libido is a reflection of the deeper conversations our bodies have with us, often whispering through the myriad balances and imbalances within us. Understanding this connection can be transformative. Physical health encompasses hormonal balance, cardiovascular efficiency, and even immune function, each playing its part in how desire is kindled or quelled. Hormones, like oestrogen and testosterone, serve as key players, orchestrating the symphony of desire, yet they can be influenced by a range of factors, such as stress or illness. Medications and chronic conditions may also cast shadows, adding complexity to the journey of rekindling libido. The pathway to desire isn't solely paved by addressing one health aspect; it's an invitation to holistically nurture your body. This begins with listening to its needs, respecting its limits, and understanding its capabilities. Empowering yourself with this knowledge is the first step towards reigniting your passion, fostering not just better physical health, but a deeper connection to your desire. As you explore these insights, remember that your journey is uniquely yours, holding the promise of rediscovery and vitality.

The Role of Hormones

In the complex tapestry of factors affecting libido, hormones are among the most pivotal yet often misunderstood players. To understand how these biochemical messengers impact sexual desire, it's important to explore their intricate influence over both the body and mind.

Hormones are essentially chemical signals that flow through your bloodstream, orchestrating a multitude of bodily functions. They affect mood, energy levels, and yes, libido. In women, the key hormones linked to sexual desire include estrogen, progesterone, and testosterone. While traditionally not the first to come to mind when considering female biology, testosterone plays a significant, albeit nuanced, role in female libido.

The hormonal cycle of menstruating women is marked by fluctuations in estrogen and progesterone levels. These shifts can have pronounced effects on sexual desire. Many women experience heightened libido around ovulation when estrogen peaks. The body, attuned to its reproductive rhythm, often signals readiness through increased desire. Yet, this experience is not universal. Some may find that the premenstrual dip in estrogen and rise in progesterone leads to irritability or mood swings, dampening sexual interest.

Transitioning into the perimenopausal and menopausal phases marks another dramatic hormonal shift. During this time, estrogen levels drop significantly, potentially leading to symptoms like vaginal dryness and discomfort during intercourse. Such physical changes can discourage sexual activity, contributing to a decline in libido. However, understanding the physiological underpinnings, women can take steps to address and even counteract these effects.

Testosterone, though commonly associated with male biology, is produced in women's bodies too, albeit in smaller quantities. It's crucial for maintaining sexual desire. Women with low levels of this hormone might experience a notable decrease in libido, while a balanced level can enhance arousal and sexual satisfaction. This points to the importance of considering testosterone levels when exploring causes of low libido in women.

On the journey to understanding hormones, it's also necessary to acknowledge how external factors can influence these internal forces. Stress, lack of sleep, and poor nutrition can all wreak havoc on hormonal balance, indirectly impacting libido. Chronic stress can increase cortisol levels, which in turn may suppress estrogen and testosterone production. This hormonal disruption not only affects desire but can also impact overall well-being.

Moreover, certain medical conditions and medications can also negatively affect hormonal balance. Conditions like polycystic ovary syndrome (PCOS) or thyroid disorders can significantly alter hormonal levels, impacting libido. An understanding of these conditions can equip women with the tools needed to seek appropriate medical advice.

Many women have turned to solutions such as hormonal replacement therapy (HRT) to manage symptoms related to menopause or hormonal imbalances. It's crucial, however, to approach this with caution and thorough consultation with a healthcare professional. The potential benefits, such as increased vagina lubrication and a return of sexual desire, need to be weighed against the risks and side effects.

What cannot be overstated is the personal nature of hormonal influence. Each woman's hormonal landscape is uniquely her own, shaped by genetics, lifestyle, and health. This makes a one-size-fits-all approach insufficient. What's essential is a tailored understanding that takes personal health narratives into account.

While the physiological effects of hormones on libido are undeniably significant, the emotional and relational aspects that intertwine with hormonal influences should not be overlooked. Hormones can sway mood and perception, impacting how one engages with a partner. Recognising this interconnectedness can foster compassion and understanding within relationships, paving the way for enhanced intimacy.

As we navigate this compelling subject, it's important to remember that there's no definitive 'right' level of libido. It's an individual journey, deeply tied to one's sense of self and personal relationships. Armed with knowledge about hormonal influences, women can gain insights into their bodies, allowing them to make informed choices and pursue a fulfilling sexual life.

In this understanding of hormones lies empowerment. By recognising the subtleties of how these chemical messengers operate, you can become your own advocate, making decisions that align with your desires and well-being. Liberation from societal pressures and misconceptions about female desire begins with informed awareness and continues through compassionate self-care.

In closing, appreciating the role of hormones in shaping libido equips women with a vital piece of the puzzle in reclaiming their sexual identity. Hormonal influences on libido are significant, but they're only one part of a broader tapestry of factors. With this understanding, you have the power to navigate your journey towards fulfilling sexual health with confidence and clarity.

Impact of Medications

When it comes to understanding the multifaceted nature of low libido, recognising the impact of medications is crucial. Various medications can directly and indirectly influence sexual desire, making it important for women to be aware of how their prescriptions might be affecting them. Modern medicine offers remarkable benefits, but it isn't without side effects. Some of these can inadvertently dampen sexual desire, adding another layer of complexity to the challenges many women face.

Many commonly prescribed medications have a known association with reduced libido. Antidepressants, particularly selective serotonin reuptake inhibitors (SSRIs), are a prominent example. While these medications play an essential role in managing depression and anxiety, they also affect neurotransmitters in the brain, which can lead to decreased sexual desire. It's a delicate balance between mental health management and maintaining a fulfilling sex life. Open communication with healthcare providers about these side effects can be pivotal in finding a solution.

Aside from antidepressants, there is a slew of other medications that can have similar impacts. Blood pressure medications, particularly beta-blockers, have been noted to cause fatigue and diminish interest in sexual activities. Similarly, certain anti-seizure medications and mood stabilisers can also reduce libido. It's fascinating how the chemistry in our brains and bodies interacts, revealing the interconnectedness of different aspects of health.

For women using hormonal contraceptives, there can be additional complications. While these are designed to manage reproductive health, some users report alterations in their libido. The hormonal changes introduced by these contraceptives might not just be about controlling pregnancy risk but can also bring about unforeseen changes in sexual desire. It's a paradox that something so integrated into women's health can also be a culprit in libido challenges.

It doesn't end there. Certain medications used to treat chronic health conditions can impact libido as well. For instance, medications for arthritis or muscle pain can lead to fatigue, which indirectly makes sexual intimacy less appealing. Additionally, medications meant to regulate blood glucose in diabetes treatments might affect energy levels and mood, both of which are crucial in nurturing a healthy sexual appetite.

The interplay between a woman's physical health and libido is deeply personal and dynamic. Each medication comes with a different set of potential impacts, and responses can vary widely among individuals. What one woman experiences might be completely different from another. This variance highlights the need for personalised medical care and the importance of advocating for oneself when discussing treatment plans with healthcare professionals.

Holistic approaches must be considered when medications begin impacting sexual health. Lifestyle adjustments, mental health therapies, and alternative treatments can complement or even mitigate the effects of certain medications. For instance, incorporating mindfulness and stress reduction techniques can help counteract the libido-dampening side effects experienced with some medications. Building a supportive network can provide emotional backing, further aiding in managing these complexities.

It's essential to remember that women have the right to both mental health and a fulfilling sexual life without having to choose between the two. Open dialogue with healthcare providers is a vital part of finding a balance. Physicians can often recommend adjustments, whether it's changing doses or trying different medications, to help minimise side effects while maintaining overall well-being.

Women also benefit from understanding that they're not alone in this struggle. Many experience these medication-induced libido changes, and sharing experiences or seeking support from networks or groups can be empowering. Building a community around discussions of sexual health is not only reassuring but can provide insights that individual experiences might not reveal.

In conclusion, medications play a crucial role in women's lives but recognising their potential impact on libido is important for making informed health decisions. Women deserve to live without the shadow of low libido overshadowing their joys. By understanding how treatments interact with our desires, alongside open communication with healthcare professionals, there's hope for a comprehensive approach to managing both health and libido amicably.

Chapter 6:
Relationship Dynamics

Relationship dynamics can significantly shape a woman's libido, weaving a complex tapestry of intimacy, communication, and emotional connection. It's vital to cultivate an open, empathetic dialogue with your partner, as this forms the cornerstone of addressing any friction that might dampen desire. Conversations around intimacy aren't just about voicing needs—they involve actively listening and understanding each other's emotional landscapes. By fostering a safe space where both partners can express vulnerabilities without judgment, you're laying the groundwork for deeper intimacy. Conflict, while sometimes inevitable, doesn't have to erode your connection; instead, it can be an opportunity to grow closer when navigated with compassion and patience. Remember, every relationship is different, and finding your rhythm requires both time and mutual effort, but the rewards are a more connected, supportive partnership where desire naturally thrives.

Communication with Your Partner

In examining the intricate dance of maintaining and nurturing romantic relationships, particularly when facing challenges like low libido, communication emerges as a crucial element. It's not merely the act of talking, but the expression of thoughts, feelings, and desires in a way that's both honest and kind. Enhancing your communication with your partner may be pivotal in addressing the drop in libido. It can act as a bridge—connecting the physical, emotional, and psychological aspects of your relationship.

Every relationship encounters its unique set of hurdles. At times, declining libido may seem like a vast chasm between partners, but addressing this openly can lead to a profound understanding of each other's needs. The cornerstone of productive communication isn't just the words spoken, but the mutual respect and empathy shared. Open conversations foster a safe space where partners can genuinely express their desires and fears without the looming threat of judgement or resentment.

When talking about sensitive subjects like libido, it might be useful to approach the conversation with empathy and patience. Recognizing the vulnerability involved is essential. Both partners need to feel heard and understood. Sometimes, it's easy to assume that because someone has been with their partner for a significant time, they instinctively know each other. However, assumptions can be misleading. Love languages and sexual appetites evolve, making it vital to frequently check in with each other.

A common myth suggests that sexual desire should be inherently spontaneous and constant, yet reality paints a different picture. Desire ebbs and flows. Embracing this fluidity rather than resisting it can be beneficial. If you're experiencing a dip, it might not necessarily indicate a lack of love or attraction. Instead, it could highlight an opportunity for growth and understanding within your relationship dynamic.

Begin these conversations in a setting that feels safe and neutral. A quiet evening at home may provide the comfort needed to broach such intimate topics. Setting the tone is vital. Frame the discussion as a team effort rather than a confrontation. Phrases like "I feel" or "I've noticed" open the door to discussion without assigning blame. Instead of accusing your partner of inadequacies, share your personal experiences and insights. This approach helps in fostering collaboration and unity.

Remember, timing can play a pivotal role. Attempting to have deep conversations when emotions are high may not lead to an effective dialogue. Choose a time when both of you are calm and receptive. In tandem with timing, active listening is paramount. Listening might seem simple, yet it requires courage and focus to truly absorb what the other is conveying without jumping in with preconceptions or solutions.

It's equally important to express gratitude and acknowledge the efforts your partner makes, no matter how small. Positive reinforcement can nurture a more accepting and loving atmosphere. When partners feel appreciated, they're more likely to reciprocate, creating a cycle of positivity and mutual support.

Moreover, as daunting as it may sound, discussing sexual fantasies or preferences can reignite passion. These conversations pave the way for better understanding your partner's deepest desires. They also present a space to explore previously unconsidered avenues of intimacy. Sharing fantasies requires a certain level of openness and vulnerability, yet the rewards of connecting on this level can be profound.

Occasionally, words might fail to capture the depth of emotions. In such instances, non-verbal communication can offer subtle yet effective tools. Simple gestures or shifts in body language often communicate more than words ever could. Holding hands, maintaining eye contact, or offering a reassuring touch can convey support and solidarity, reminding each other of the partnership's strength.

In scenarios where conversations seem to falter or tensions rise, it may be beneficial to introduce professional guidance. Counsellors have the skills to mediate conversations, offering insightful perspectives and exercises to improve communication. They can provide the tools necessary to tackle seemingly insurmountable issues, transforming challenges into opportunities for growth.

It's worth noting that patience is key. Transformation doesn't occur overnight. Communication is a journey rather than a destination. With continued effort and understanding, the strains of low libido can become less burdensome, revealing a relationship that's enriched and deepened by the trials faced together.

Ultimately, effective communication with your partner is a life skill. Its benefits extend beyond the bedroom, enhancing trust, empathy, and connection in all aspects of your shared life. Through this ongoing dialogue, you can confront low libido collectively, turning it into a step towards an even more intimate and fulfilling relationship.

Addressing Conflict and Intimacy

In every relationship, harmony and discord dance hand in hand. The way we address conflict has a tremendous impact on intimacy. When left unchecked, unresolved disputes can build walls between partners, diminishing desire and closing doors to closeness. Yet, when navigated with care and understanding, these very conflicts can be seeds of deeper connection and more meaningful experiences of intimacy.

At the heart of any conflict is a need—an unmet expectation or a boundary that's been crossed. Recognising this transforms conflict from a battleground into an opportunity for dialogue and understanding. It's not merely about addressing the immediate issue; it's about delving deeper to truly understand ourselves and our partners. By doing so, we open pathways to increased intimacy. Intimacy thrives not in the absence of conflict but in the shared journey of navigating through it.

The first step in addressing conflict is communication. Conversation is indispensable when it comes to resolving misunderstandings or disagreements. Expressing feelings openly without judgment fosters an environment where both partners can be heard and understood. Remember, it's not just about telling your side of the story; listening to your partner's perspective is equally crucial. This exchange builds trust, which is the cornerstone of intimacy.

Effective communication in times of conflict calls for empathy. Empathise with your partner's feelings and experiences. It might take a conscious effort to pause and consider their viewpoint, especially when emotions are running high. Yet, it's a powerful tool. When we feel genuinely understood, barriers break down, allowing us to connect on a deeper, more meaningful level.

Another essential component is forgiveness. Holding onto past grievances creates emotional distance, whereas forgiveness clears the way for renewed intimacy. It's not about excusing past mistakes but releasing their grip on your present relationship. Through forgiveness, you allow healing and invite warmth back into your partnership.

Conflict often shines a spotlight on our vulnerabilities. These moments, albeit uncomfortable, provide opportunities to share and explore parts of ourselves we may have kept hidden. Sharing vulnerabilities can be daunting, but it also nurtures genuine intimacy and closeness. By showing our true selves to our partners and them doing the same, we create safe spaces for emotional and physical connection.

Boundaries play a pivotal role in maintaining a healthy dynamic. Clear boundaries help prevent conflict from escalating and provide each partner with a sense of security within the relationship. Establishing these boundaries requires honest conversation about personal limits and expectations. Honour each other's boundaries, and you're likely to find that conflict becomes less threatening and intimacy more accessible.

It's important not to lose sight of individual needs amid a relationship. While the focus may be on the partnership, each person still has unique desires and aspirations. Ensuring that these are not neglected can prevent the build-up of resentment—a common trigger for conflict. Encouraging personal fulfilment can actually strengthen the bond between partners, leading to a more vibrant and connecting intimacy.

Conflict can also serve as a catalyst for growth. Each disagreement provides an opportunity to learn and adapt, leading to stronger relational skills and deeper understanding. Seeing conflict as a growth opportunity rather than a threat can inspire more constructive approaches to resolving differences. This shift in perspective can transform conflict from a source of stress into a platform for enhancing intimacy.

Don't shy away from seeking professional help if conflicts seem insurmountable. Sometimes, talking to a relationship counsellor introduces new perspectives and strategies that might not be apparent when caught up in the emotion of conflict. Professional guidance can provide valuable insights and equip you with tools to maintain both peace and intimacy in your relationship.

Ultimately, addressing conflict and nurturing intimacy boil down to shared commitment. A conscious and collective decision to work through challenges together reinforces the foundation of your relationship. This commitment ensures that both partners are invested in finding solutions and fostering a connection that supports deeper intimacy.

As you navigate these dynamics, remember that conflict is an inevitable part of life. It's how we choose to engage with and resolve these conflicts that shapes the quality of our relationships. By approaching conflicts as opportunities for learning, growth, and connection, intimacy no longer becomes a distant goal but an ongoing journey—with each step, you're deepening the bond between yourself and your partner.

Chapter 7:
Rediscovering Your Body

In the journey towards rekindling desire, rediscovering your body is a deeply personal exploration that invites you to embrace your unique physicality as an empowering ally. This chapter encourages you to acknowledge and celebrate the evolution of your body, recognising that each change brings with it a story of resilience and grace. It's about shifting the narrative from one of criticism to one of curiosity, allowing you to enhance body confidence in a way that feels authentic and affirming. By reconnecting with your senses and tapping into the intrinsic pleasure that your body can offer, you'll find a renewed sense of intimacy with yourself. This isn't just about learning to love your reflection; it's about understanding that your body is a gateway to a deeper connection with your desires, unfolding new layers of intimacy ready to be explored and celebrated. Embrace this newfound confidence as a foundation for building a fulfilling, passionate life where desire flourishes naturally and joyfully.

Embracing Physical Change

When it comes to intimacy, recognising and embracing the changes our bodies undergo is a significant component of rediscovering one's sexual self. Women's bodies evolve throughout their lives, influenced by a multitude of factors such as age, childbirth, hormonal shifts, and even the delicate dance with stress and lifestyle dynamics. Adapting to these changes can feel daunting—sometimes even as an admittance of vulnerability—but it can also be an empowering journey, an invitation to redefine your relationship with your body and, ultimately, your desire.

As we age, physical changes might seem to signal an unwelcome shift in our sexuality. However, it's crucial to acknowledge that change doesn't necessarily mean decline. Instead, it can open new doors to pleasure and understanding that may have been overlooked in younger years. Embracing bodily transformation begins with acceptance. The softness of your skin, the slight rounding of your belly, and the silvering of your hair are all narratives, stories your body has lived and tells every day.

These physical changes can inspire a deeper appreciation for your body and what it's capable of, urging you to listen more closely to its needs and desires. A shift in perspective—from seeing your body as static and unchanging to a dynamic, evolving entity—can transform how you approach sexual intimacy. This isn't merely a mental exercise; it's a whole-hearted embrace of yourself, quirks and all, which naturally enhances your libido, liberating you from unrealistic societal expectations of perpetual youth.

One practical approach to embracing physical change is through body positivity and self-care rituals. This might mean spending a few moments in the morning to appreciate your reflection. It could involve indulging in a beauty regime not for the result, but for the process—a deliberate act of self-love. Honour your body with nourishing foods and gentle movement. These practices help nurture a connection with oneself that can reignite sexual desire, shifting focus from what the body looks like to what it feels like, increasing both self-confidence and sexual responsiveness.

As you navigate these changes, communicating with your partner about your physical transformation and its impacts on your intimacy can be empowering. Engage in open, honest discussions about your experiences. Sharing these intimate insights not only fosters an understanding environment but also encourages your partner to actively participate in the journey alongside you. Such collaborations in intimacy can lead to a more profound and fulfilling sexual connection, characterised by shared exploration and mutual discovery.

It's equally important to explore and potentially embrace any medical interventions that might support these transitions, be it through nutritional supplements or medical advice. Hormonal shifts, such as those experienced during menopause or following childbirth, can significantly impact libido and intimacy. Consulting healthcare professionals to better understand the nuances of these changes can enable you to adapt and make informed choices that best suit your lifestyle and enhance your sexual health.

Mindfulness practices can also play a pivotal role. Engaging with your body and desires in the present moment—without judgement—can help you become more attuned to the subtle shifts and new sensations that come with physical change. Mindfulness helps in breaking free from a past version of the self, offering a fresh palette for painting the new canvas of your sexual identity.

Lastly, let's not forget the power of sexual exploration as a tool for embracing physical change. Masturbation and self-exploration can serve as essential practices for understanding newly emerging sensations and desires in an evolving body. Adjusting these practices to align with bodily changes can help you maintain a satisfying sexual self-awareness. It's an intimate conversation with the self that invites curiosity and compassion.

Physical change, therefore, doesn't have to be met with resistance or reluctance. Instead, it can be an opportunity for growth and transformation. Rediscovering the sensual and sexual power within these changes allows you to move forward with confidence, elevating intimacy and reinforcing your sense of self-worth. Embrace this new chapter not just as a transition but as an exciting entry point into deeper self-discovery and empowerment.

Enhancing Body Confidence

Rediscovering your body is more than just acknowledging its physical existence; it's about celebrating its uniqueness and building a compassionate relationship with it. Enhancing body confidence plays a crucial role in this journey. When you feel good about how you look, your sense of self-worth and attractiveness can dramatically increase, positively impacting your libido. It's not about aspiring to fit into societal standards, but about cherishing the body you have. Appreciating your body for its strengths, its endurance, and its beauty can transform how you perceive yourself and, ultimately, how you interact intimately with your partner.

To begin enhancing body confidence, it's essential to shift the focus from perceived flaws to the unique attributes that make you, you. Take time to reflect on what your body allows you to do: it carries you through the world, lets you experience every taste and touch, and gives you the capability to connect deeply with another person. Emphasising these aspects can foster a sense of gratitude for your body, which is fundamental in building confidence. By recognising and celebrating these aspects, you reinforce positive self-esteem and nurture an intimate appreciation and acceptance of your form.

Creating rituals that celebrate your body can be an incredibly transformative practice. Incorporate simple and affirming rituals into your daily routine. This might include a nurturing skincare routine, mindful movement like yoga or dancing, or even soaking in a warm bath, savouring the sensation of water on your skin. These practices are not merely acts of self-care, but declarations of your worth. They remind you that your body is deserving of care and adoration. They allow you to connect with your physical self in a gentle, affirming way, and in doing so, they help establish a deeper feeling of body confidence.

A personal style that enhances your body confidence is another effective tool in your arsenal. Dressing in a way that expresses who you are can shift your perception of your body. Choose clothes that fit well, feel good, and make you stand tall. When you wear something that you love and that feels right for you, it can elevate your mood and provide a powerful boost to your self-assurance. It's not about dressing to impress others, but about dressing to express the beautiful, unique person you are.

The language you use when talking about your body is also significant. Pay attention to your inner dialogue. Replace critical self-talk with supportive, loving affirmations. Focus on the features you admire, and speak kindly about your perceived imperfections. Phrases like "I appreciate my strong legs" or "I love my radiant smile" can reshape the way you see yourself. Language is powerful; by consciously deciding to speak positively, you can transform your perception of your body from a point of insecurity to a source of confidence.

Opening yourself up to body positivity involves challenging and then changing harmful societal norms and biases, both personally and communally. It's essential to surround yourself with messages and influences that promote diverse representations of beauty. This might mean curating your social media feeds to include a wide array of body types, or choosing books and media that reflect varied narratives about beauty and self-worth. Watching your inner media diet can help you pivot towards acceptance and pride in your own body.

Another aspect worth considering is the role of physical activity in enhancing body confidence. It's not solely about achieving an ideal physique. Engaging in physical activity, be it running, swimming, or stretching, connects you to your body's capability and strength. This connection is empowering. It reinforces the recognition that your body is a source of strength, endurance, and vitality. Moreover, as you consistently engage in physical activities, your body may change, and feeling stronger and more agile can naturally boost how you perceive your body.

When nurturing body confidence, it's important to also address the emotional ties linked to body image. Body confidence can sometimes waver based on insecurities or past experiences. Conversations with a therapist or counsellor about body image concerns might be beneficial. Such dialogues can uncover underlying issues, address deep-seated beliefs, and provide tools for building a healthier perception of yourself. These emotional explorations can lead you to embrace your body with renewed empathy, understanding, and love.

A community of support can have a profound effect on how you see your body. Engaging with groups or friends who celebrate body positivity and encourage open and accepting dialogue about body image can be a refreshing and nurturing experience. These interactions provide reassurance that you're not alone in your struggles, and they offer a platform for sharing tips, encouragement, and positivity. Being part of such a community reminds you of the collective journey towards self-love and eradicates the perceived norms that can weigh down on body confidence.

Lastly, recognising that body confidence is an evolving journey rather than a destination is crucial. Your perception of your body might change with time, experiences, and reflections, and that's perfectly normal. Embrace this fluidity as part of your life. Celebrate the small victories, be patient with the setbacks, and consistently reaffirm your worth and beauty. Enhancing body confidence is not about reaching a final point of acceptance, but rather about fostering a constant state of appreciation and love for the body you inhabit now and in the time to come.

Chapter 8:
Lifestyle Changes for Libido

Embracing lifestyle changes can be a powerful step in reigniting your libido and fostering a deeper connection with your partner. It's not just about altering habits but adopting a holistic approach that nurtures both mind and body. Imagine how a well-balanced diet, rich in nutrients, can subtly enhance your desire, while regular exercise stimulates not only the body but invigorates the intimate journey with newfound vitality. Each lifestyle choice, from the nourishing foods you consume to the energy-boosting workouts you embrace, plays a pivotal role in enhancing sexual health. Remember, these aren't mere tasks but investments in your well-being, layering in health benefits that naturally ripple into your sexual experiences. By weaving these small yet impactful changes into daily life, you're not only paving the way to a renewed libido but enriching your entire existence with vibrancy and a deeper sense of fulfilment.

Nutrition and Its Impact on Desire

Nutrition plays an integral role in many aspects of our lives, and sexual health is no exception. The food we consume doesn't just have a bearing on our physical health; it significantly influences our emotional and psychological well-being, both of which are critical in maintaining a healthy libido. For women experiencing low desire, understanding the link between nutrition and libido can open new pathways to rekindle that spark.

A balanced diet rich in essential nutrients can enhance overall health and well-being, which in turn can lead to a positive impact on sexual desire. Certain foods are known to support hormone production, and hormones play a critical role in sexual function. For instance, zinc and omega-3 fatty acids are essential for the production of testosterone, a hormone present in both men and women that is closely tied to sexual desire. Oysters, fatty fish, and pumpkin seeds are excellent dietary sources of these nutrients.

Moreover, maintaining good cardiovascular health through a nutritious diet can improve blood flow, which is crucial for sexual arousal. Foods that support heart health, like leafy greens, berries, and nuts, can promote better circulation. Improved blood flow means increased sensitivity and responsiveness, enhancing sexual experiences.

In addition to the physical benefits, nutrition has a profound effect on mood and energy levels. A diet rich in vitamins B and D, magnesium, and low in sugars and processed foods can help stabilise mood fluctuations and boost energy levels. When you feel energised and emotionally balanced, you're more likely to have a healthy and active sex drive. Foods like whole grains, dark chocolate, and lentils can contribute to this well-being.

It's important to understand the negative impact certain foods and substances can have on libido. Excessive alcohol, for instance, is known to dampen sexual desire by altering hormone levels and affecting the nervous system. Similarly, diets high in processed foods and sugar can lead to weight gain and decreased energy, both of which may impact self-esteem and libido. Managing a healthy, balanced diet while moderating alcohol consumption can be crucial steps towards improving desire.

Caffeine intake warrants consideration too. While moderate consumption might have a temporary energising effect, excessive caffeine can lead to anxiety and disrupted sleep—both significant libido dampeners. Finding a balance and choosing sources such as green tea, with its health benefits, or simply ensuring you stay within recommended limits, can mitigate these negative effects.

Fostering a healthy relationship with food involves listening to your body's needs and responding with mindfulness and balance. Engaging in mindful eating practices can enhance your bodily awareness, creating a deeper connection to how different foods affect not just your body, but your mind too. Be present during meals, savour your food, and pay attention to how it makes you feel both immediately and over time.

For women facing low libido, exploring nutrition as a supportive tool is an empowering choice. It opens up possibilities for making active decisions that can influence desire and sexual experience positively. With every nourishing bite, you're not just feeding your body but also fuelling the potential for genuine connection and desire.

Ultimately, it's important to remember that everyone's body is different, and what works for one person may not work for another. Paying attention to what your body needs and consulting healthcare professionals or nutritionists can guide you in finding what works best for you. Creating an eating plan that supports your overall health and libido is an individual journey, and it's a powerful form of self-care.

This section of the book is dedicated to helping you harness the power of nutrition as part of a broader strategy to enhance your libido. Remember, improving your sexual health and desire requires a holistic approach, and making informed dietary choices is a key component on that path to sexual wellness. Combining these insights with other lifestyle modifications, like exercise and mindfulness, which will be explored in subsequent sections, can be transformative.

Exercise for Sexual Health

When we think about exercise, the usual suspects that come to mind are weight loss, muscle gain, or cardiovascular health. But have you ever considered exercise as an invigorating elixir for your sexual health? Physical activity plays a pivotal role not only in keeping our bodies fit but also in nurturing a vibrant libido. It's no secret that a well-exercised body is a happy body, and this joy often translates into a more fulfilling sexual life.

Physical activity enhances the body's natural ability to produce endorphins, those delightful chemicals that elevate our mood and reduce stress. For women experiencing low libido, exercise can serve as a natural antidote to stress and anxiety, two significant blockers of sexual desire. Imagine the freedom that comes from shedding the worries of the day and immersing yourself in the sheer vitality of movement. This liberation often leads to an enhanced connection with one's physical self, paving the way for increased sexual desire.

Strength and endurance exercises are not just about chiselling abs or lifting more weight. They carve out confidence—a subtle yet potent aphrodisiac. When you feel strong in your body, you feel capable and confident, sensations that make the dance of intimacy not only possible but eagerly anticipated. Ladies, imagine walking into the bedroom not just knowing but feeling that you're capable of whatever the moment calls for. That's the power of exercise at work.

It's important not to overlook the wonders of flexibility and balance exercises. Practices like yoga and Pilates don't just improve your range of motion; they awaken a deeper awareness of your body. This heightened physical consciousness can translate into better sexual performance and satisfaction. Yoga, in particular, is known for its emphasis on mindful breathing and relaxation, tools that can be extrapolated to enhance a sexual encounter. Imagine the depth and richness of an intimate moment amplified because you're fully present, aware of each nuanced sensation.

Various forms of exercise can cater to improving your sexual health in different ways. Cardiovascular activities, like brisk walking, swimming, or dancing, improve circulation, which is vital for sexual arousal in women. Better circulation means more blood flow to your genitals, heightening sensitivity and overall pleasure. Picture this: the simple joy of a brisk evening walk not only keeps your heart healthy but also primes your body for intimacy later on.

It's not just about the physical benefits; exercise also fosters a mental resilience that is crucial for sexual wellbeing. Regular physical activity boosts self-esteem and body image, both of which are intimately tied to a healthy libido. When you're engaged in regular exercise, you begin to shift focus from how your body looks to what it can do—a powerful shift that empowers you in the realm of sexual confidence.

Additionally, exercise can be a thrilling shared activity with your partner, enhancing your bond outside the confines of a bedroom. Think of a dance class or a weekend hike. These activities allow couples to connect in playful and novel settings, building intimacy through shared experiences and laughter. It's a reminder that sexual health encompasses more than just the act—it involves the entire tapestry of your relationship.

Resistance training and exercises targeting the core can improve your pelvic floor muscles, which play a crucial role in sexual function and satisfaction. A strong pelvic floor can enhance pleasure and intensify orgasms, adding an element of excitement and anticipation to your intimate life. Simple Kegel exercises can be incorporated into your daily routine, subtly enhancing your sexual health over time without the need for a gym session.

Often, the biggest step is just getting started. The thought of exercise, especially if it's been a while, can feel daunting. Start small. Perhaps a gentle yoga session or a short walk around the neighbourhood. Give yourself permission to find joy in movement, allowing it to become a cherished part of your daily life rather than a chore. It's through these small steps that transformation occurs—not just in your fitness level, but in your sexual health as well.

Lastly, remember that physical activity needs to be something you enjoy. If you're forcing yourself into exercise routines that don't excite or energise you, then it's time for a change. Explore various forms of movement until you find what lights you up, be it dancing, cycling, or even martial arts. The key is to integrate movement into your lifestyle in a way that feels authentic and enjoyable for you.

In conclusion, exercise is more than just a path to physical fitness; it's a doorway to enhancing your sexual health. By embracing a routine that incorporates flexibility, strength, and cardiovascular exercises, you not only promote a healthy libido but also cultivate a sense of empowerment in your sexual life. As you continue to explore and rediscover your body's capabilities, you'll find that the benefits extend far beyond the physical, nurturing a deeper connection to your mind, body, and partner.

Chapter 9:
Mindfulness and Desire

In a world buzzing with distractions and endless to-do lists, finding the path to rekindling sexual desire might seem daunting. However, embracing mindfulness can be a transformative approach to reconnecting with your desires. This chapter delves into the art of being present—where physical intimacy becomes a shared moment unclouded by past grievances or future anxieties. Mindfulness invites you to experience touch, whispers, and warmth in their most authentic forms, rekindling a visceral connection and mutual awareness with your partner. By practising mindful presence during intimate moments, you can forge a deeper, more meaningful bond that nourishes both desire and emotional intimacy. A mindful approach allows you to let go of self-judgement and societal pressures, focusing instead on the beauty of the present moment, where genuine connection can thrive. As you explore these techniques, you're not just maintaining physical intimacy; you're nurturing a space where desire can blossom naturally and passionately, leading to a fulfilling sexual life.

Practising Presence in Intimacy

In today's fast-paced world, many aspects of our lives demand our attention almost constantly. Whether it's work, family, or social commitments, the noise can be overwhelming and the chaos all-consuming. Amidst this, the idea of practising presence in intimacy becomes not just a beneficial practice but a vital one. For women seeking to rekindle desire, cultivating a mindful state during intimate moments can prove transformative. Intimacy requires focus, a quality often eroded by our tendency to multitask or dwell on past worries and future concerns.

Being present with a partner isn't just about physical presence. It's about tuning in emotionally and mentally, fully engaging with the sensations, emotions, and experiences that arise. Such presence allows us to truly connect, not only with our partner but also with ourselves. This connection can awaken dormant desires and amplify the satisfaction derived from intimate interactions.

The journey towards mindfulness in intimate settings begins with self-awareness. Understanding one's own mind and body is a precursor to experiencing deeper connection. It involves acknowledging thoughts and feelings without judgment. For many women, sexual moments, instead of being instances of pleasure, might bring anxieties or insecurities to the fore. These feelings are valid, but observing them without letting them overshadow the moment can be liberating. Through practice, it becomes possible to acknowledge a wandering mind and gently steer it back to the present.

Imagine involving all your senses to amplify your engagement. The smells, sounds, tastes, and touches during intimacy are doorways to staying present. Each sensation is an opportunity to deepen awareness. The softness of skin, the rhythm of a heartbeat, or even the quiet moments of shared stillness can tether you back to the now. Developing an appreciation for these subtle nuances requires practice, but the rewards—heightened pleasure and connection—are worth the effort.

Mindfulness isn't just an individual practice; it thrives in shared experiences. Communication plays a pivotal role in voicing your needs and understanding your partner's, ensuring that both parties feel valued and respected. By sharing intentions, couples can create a more open and accepting environment. This mutual understanding celebrates the uniqueness of each moment, fostering a bond that's both passionate and gentle.

Incorporating mindful practices can begin in simple, non-intimate settings. Activities like shared breathing exercises or mindful walks can encourage partners to be more in tune with one another. Such routines outside of intimate moments nurture a habit of presence that naturally extends to more private encounters.

Consider exploring guided mindfulness exercises designed to enhance intimacy. These may include practices focusing on synchronised breathing, where the rhythm of breaths becomes a bridge connecting the inner worlds of two individuals. Such exercises not only facilitate physical closeness but also promote emotional transparency and trust.

The power of touch, although simple, is profound. Mindful touch is intentional; it's about being fully engrossed in the sensations and emotions it provokes. Whether through the gentlest caress or a more vigorous embrace, mindful touch encourages a symphonic engagement of the senses, coaxing the mind to let go of distractions and provide presence with full attention.

Building this skill requires patience, as much with oneself as with one's partner. It may feel awkward at first, or even frustrating, when the mind refuses to remain tethered to the present. That's normal. Like any worthwhile practice, mastering presence in intimacy takes dedication and an open mind. Encouragement and persistence pave the road to greater fulfillment.

Embracing vulnerability is another cornerstone of mindful intimacy. It allows both partners to see and be seen as they are: genuine, honest, and open-hearted. This authenticity can dismantle barriers and misconceptions that often arise from fear or doubt. By cultivating vulnerability, couples engage in a dance of trust, a sacred exchange that strengthens bonds and nurtures desire.

Ultimately, practising presence in intimate moments is about letting go of expectations. It's about allowing what is to emerge organically, welcoming whatever arises with kindness and curiosity. This acceptance makes space for discovery—not only in terms of shared joy but also in understanding and compassion toward oneself and one's partner.

In the ebb and flow of life, mindful intimacy acts as a harbour, a sanctuary where desires aren't rushed or forced but rediscovered and tenderly embraced. Presence turns fleeting moments into meaningful, lasting impressions, weaving a tapestry of love and connection that nourishes the soul.

So, as you step into this exploration, remember that mindfulness in intimacy isn't a destination but a journey—a beautiful unfolding that invites more depth, pleasure, and resilience into your life. Let this practice be a reminder of the innate power of presence to transform the ordinary into the extraordinary.

Techniques for Mindful Connection

As we delve deeper into the relationship between mindfulness and desire, it becomes evident that cultivating a mindful approach to intimacy can profoundly impact one's sexual experience. Mindfulness, in this context, is all about being present, attentive, and receptive to both your own sensations and those of your partner. It isn't a quick fix, but rather a journey—one that gradually transforms intimacy into a more fulfilling encounter.

One of the most effective techniques for fostering mindful connection is through breath awareness. Focusing on your breath during intimate moments can anchor you in the present. By tuning into the natural rhythm of inhalations and exhalations, you bring your awareness away from distractions and closer to your immediate experience. This simple act can create a sense of calm, reducing anxiety and allowing you to be more engaged.

Consider integrating intentional touch into your practice of mindful connection. This involves exploring your own body—or your partner's—with a sense of purpose. Instead of going through the motions, pay close attention to what feels pleasurable. Is your skin tingling? Are there goosebumps? Take note of these sensations and allow them to guide your movements. By doing so, you're not just engaging in physical contact but also deepening the emotional and sensual bond you share.

Moreover, mindful connection isn't just about the physical aspects of intimacy. Emotional presence plays a crucial role. Listening with empathy and expressing your feelings with authenticity can open pathways to deeper connection. Engage in honest conversations about desires, boundaries, and curiosities without fear of judgement. This transparency paves the way for a safe space where both you and your partner feel valued and heard.

Incorporating mindfulness exercises into your daily routine can also support your journey towards deeper connection. Practices like meditation, yoga, or tai chi can heighten your bodily awareness and improve your ability to focus. These practices cultivate patience, too, which can be invaluable in intimate settings. As you become more adept at staying present in the moment, you'll likely find that this mindfulness spills over into other areas of your relationship.

Visualisation is another potent tool for mindful connection. Picture yourself in a serene environment where you feel completely at ease. Envision an experience filled with warmth, acceptance, and love. Visualisation can help in setting the mood, relieving stress, and creating a desired emotional atmosphere that encourages relaxation and openness. Let your imagination be a canvas on which you paint a fulfilling and desired intimate experience.

Try experimenting with mindful synching exercises with your partner. These can range from breathing in unison to intentional eye contact that lasts longer than usual. Such exercises can create an intimate, shared presence and enhance your emotional link. This deeper connection might startle you with its intensity, but it can also rekindle a sense of wonder and curiosity about each other.

It's worth mentioning the power of letting go of expectations. Mindfulness encourages acceptance of the present moment as it is. Instead of focusing on an end goal, immerse yourself in the journey itself. When expectations dissolve, space is created for genuine smiles, laughter, and a joyful appreciation of shared moments.

Practicing gratitude within your relationship can enhance mindful connection as well. Reflect on the aspects of your partner and the relationship that you cherish. Sharing these reflections openly can foster emotional intimacy and gratitude for each other's presence. Expressing gratitude shifts your focus onto positives, lessening the hold of external pressures or stresses.

For those who feel disconnected from their bodies or struggle with negative body image, mindfulness practices focusing on body positivity can enhance your intimate experience. Start by appreciating small things about your body, celebrating its strength, resilience, and beauty. Acknowledge its ability to experience pleasure and the joy it can bring. This recognition fosters confidence, which is key in nurturing desire and connection.

Finally, it's important to remember that mindful connection is not devoid of seriousness but should also embrace playfulness and curiosity. Explore new activities, be it dance lessons or trying new fantasies, that allow you to express this playfulness. By introducing elements of surprise and novelty, both you and your partner can embark on a journey that keeps the flame of curiosity alive, asks questions, and invites answers.

Through these techniques for mindful connection, you'll find a newfound harmony not only within yourself but also in your relationship. By consciously engaging in each interaction, you create a robust foundation for emotional and physical intimacy. When you're present and attentive, with each breath, touch, and whisper, you're choosing to nurture your desire and infuse your relationship with warmth and understanding. Embrace this journey as an invitation to connect more profoundly with your partner and yourself.

Chapter 10:
Exploring Sensuality

Embarking on the journey of exploring sensuality is like discovering a hidden facet of yourself, a unique layer that enriches your intimacy and deepens your connections. It's about awakening your senses—those delightful touchpoints that go beyond the mind and body, encapsulating the heart and soul. Imagine strolling through a lush garden: the gentle caress of a breeze, the intoxicating aroma of blooming flowers, the warm embrace of the sun—it's these subtle moments that remind us of the magic our senses can create. By nurturing your sensual awareness, you're crafting a space for desire to flourish naturally. Whether it's the silken feel of your favourite fabric against your skin or the lingering notes of a beloved melody, these experiences can revive and intensify your sensual life. As you become attuned to these sensations, not only does your desire spark, but a newfound appreciation for your body and its pleasures blossoms, inspiring a deeper connection to yourself and, in turn, with your partner. Embrace this exploration with openness and curiosity, for it's in these nuances of sensual presence that the richest intimacy is found.

Reviving Sensual Awareness

As we dive into the process of reviving sensual awareness, it's essential to understand that sensuality is distinct from sexuality. It's about engaging all five senses and becoming more attuned to the world around you. Your senses serve as a gateway to deeper intimacy, both with yourself and your partner. Personal connection with your sensuality can be a powerful factor in reigniting desire, as it allows you to enjoy the present moment more fully. Let's explore how a renewed focus on your senses can help breathe life back into your libido.

Start by creating an environment that stimulates your senses in subtle yet impactful ways. Think about the lighting, scents, and sounds that make you feel relaxed and at ease. Perhaps it's the gentle flicker of candlelight or the calming aroma of lavender. Sensual awareness begins with these small shifts. It invites you to slow down and take in each moment with intention. Consider incorporating soft fabrics into your wardrobe or environment that invite touch and comfort, further enhancing your awareness of the tactile elements of daily life. The act of being more present with your surroundings can lead to a natural increase in bodily awareness and responsiveness.

Engaging with your senses can be an empowering experience. Tune into the sounds of your favourite music and allow it to move you. Dance when you feel inspired, letting your body respond to the rhythm and beat. You might find that immersing yourself in music provides a release, an opportunity to express yourself physically and emotionally. Music can be a potent tool for reconnecting with your body and emotions, helping you to rediscover joy and pleasure. It's a reminder that sensuality doesn't have to contribute to stress or performance pressure, but can be a liberating experience where freedom and spontaneity reign.

Food is another incredible medium for examining and enhancing sensuality. Paying attention to the taste and texture of what you consume turns eating into a more gratifying experience. Savour each mouthful, allowing yourself to fully appreciate the flavours and aroma. This focused attention not only transforms eating into a pleasurable event but also teaches you to slow your pace and be present in each moment. Over time, extending this mindfulness to other facets of life, including intimacy, becomes more instinctual.

Exploration of the natural world can also serve to heighten sensual awareness. A walk in the park or spending time by the ocean provides a plethora of sensations. The feel of the sun on your skin, the sound of leaves rustling in the wind, and the fresh scent of the earth after rain can ground you, providing a sensual experience unlike any other. These experiences remind you of your connection to nature and your place within it, fostering a deeper appreciation of life and self.

Creating a journal of your experiences can support you in tracking how engaging your senses impacts your libido and overall mood. Write about each activity you've tried and the emotions or thoughts that emerged. Note the scents that bring you joy, the music that makes you feel vibrant, the tactile interactions that soothe your soul. Over time, you'll likely notice patterns and preferences that help inform which experiences to embrace more regularly, refining your journey towards a revived sensual self.

Don't be afraid to step beyond the tried and tested. Experimentation is a part of growth, and each sensory experience enriches your understanding of what brings you pleasure. Whether it's trying a new type of yoga or experimenting with essential oils, variety spices up your routine and can lead you to undiscovered aspects of your sensuality.

Practising self-compassion is equally important. Some days, the reconnection will flow naturally, and other days might require more effort. During challenging times, remember that reviving sensual awareness is a journey, not a destination. Self-criticism can impede progress, while patience and kindness towards oneself can yield more fruitful results. Embrace each step with acceptance and an open heart.

Finally, sharing this journey with a partner can enhance the experience, but it's not a necessity. Your sensual awareness is deeply personal, and coming to realise its potential can be a solo venture. However, if you're inclined, inviting a partner to join can deepen your shared connection. Engage in mutual sensory experiences—such as cooking a meal together, dancing in your living room, or simply sitting in comfortable silence—each activity offering a distinct opportunity to connect and appreciate one another's presence.

Understanding and reviving your sensual awareness can be transformative. It's a return not only to desire but also to a fuller life experience. This newfound awareness enlightens your path, enabling you to foster a more profound connection with yourself and others, and encouraging a dynamic and resilient libido.

Enhancing Sensual Experiences

Understanding and enhancing your sensual experiences can pave the way to rediscovering and embracing your innate desires. It's not just about the grand gestures or clichéd candles and wine, but the everyday moments and subtle shifts in awareness that can reignite a dulled sense of passion. Sensual experiences aren't solely about physical touch— they're about engaging all your senses in a way that makes everything a little more vibrant, a little more alive.

Imagine walking through a beautiful garden, the aroma of roses wafting around you, the sunlight filtering through the leaves and dancing on your skin, the gentle rustle of the breeze in your ear. These aren't just sensory experiences, they're opportunities to connect deeply with the world and yourself. Allowing everyday experiences to invigorate your sensuality can be incredibly empowering. It's about allowing those moments to beckon you into a world of pleasure—one where your senses are the artists painting a vivid picture of desire.

One powerful way to enhance sensual experiences is through mindful exploration of your physical self. Becoming attuned to the various textures, pressures, and rhythms that make up your sensory world can be a beautiful act of self-love and discovery. It starts with something as simple as a touch. Run your fingers through your hair, across your skin—notice how your body responds. Learn to listen to these reactions without the distraction of judgement or expectation.

Tapping into your creativity can also serve as a catalyst for sensual exploration. Creativity isn't confined to painting or music; it's the way you arrange your home, choose your clothes, or even how you approach cooking meals. Each of these activities can be transformed into a sensual expression by consciously immersing yourself in the texture, aroma, and appearance of everything around you. Engage these experiences fully and allow your senses to travel freely through your world.

Opening up to new experiences and adventures can also enhance your sensual life. We often fall into patterns that become familiar and routine, with predictability stifling the excitement necessary for desire. By venturing into the new, whether it's an art class, a culinary course or something entirely out of your comfort zone, you help break these patterns. These new experiences can stir curiosity, excitement, and anticipation—all potent aphrodisiacs for the soul.

The way you experience sensuality is not limited within the confines of your own body and mind. Invest time in creating an environment that stimulates your senses. Think about incorporating textures that you enjoy, fabrics that feel decadent against your skin, and lighting that flatters both you and your space. Use scents that lift your mood and evoke comforting or energising memories, or try something new and unusual to see how it resonates with you.

Sound, too, plays a critical role in your sensual landscape. Exploring music that resonates with your emotional and physical being can be a transformative practice. It's more than background noise; it's an entryway into emotional and physical release and a tuning fork for your moods. Whether it's the soothing strums of a guitar or the pulsing beat of a drum, let the sounds you choose elevate ordinary moments into something extraordinary.

Transforming routine tasks into sensory rituals can be both grounding and liberating, laying a foundation upon which desire can grow. Showering, for instance, can become a sanctuary: feel the water's temperature as it cascades down your body, listen to the sound it makes as it hits the surface, and observe how your skin reacts with each drop. These everyday acts can be small yet profound gestures of self-appreciation and rejuvenation.

Experimenting with sensory deprivation as a contrast can also heighten your perception of other senses. Wearing a blindfold or applying earplugs during certain activities might intensify the sensations of touch, taste, and smell, providing a new realm of possibility in how you experience pleasure. It's an intriguing paradox: by removing certain stimuli, others become impossibly clear and vivid.

Cultivating this awareness and appreciation for the senses can bring a sense of novelty and renewal. The connection to your sensual self is an ongoing dialogue, an exploration that doesn't necessitate reaching a particular goal to be enjoyable. Enhance your sensory experiences by noticing the nuances around you more frequently and inviting gratitude for the pleasure they bring.

In strengthening these connections, it's essential to communicate and share your findings and desires with your partner, should you have one. Openness about your sensory world can foster deeper emotional and physical intimacy, helping bridge the gap that low libido might have created. Partners who understand your sensory preferences are better equipped to fulfil desires and participate actively in enhancing sensual experiences.

Enhancing sensual experiences requires intention and time—an investment in self-care that's infinitely worth the effort. It's a gentle revolution against the current of stress, routine, and disconnection. It's about giving yourself permission to enjoy your body and surroundings in the fullest sense. These experiences can act as an anchor, grounding you in moments that might otherwise drift away unnoticed.

Ultimately, enhancing your sensual experiences is about finding joy and curiosity within yourself and your world. It's a journey of exploration that's boundless and ever-evolving. Reclaim that connection to your senses, and in it, discover the vibrant foundations on which your sexual desire can thrive. By embracing these experiences, you lay the groundwork for a more enriched and fulfilling sense of sexual self-awareness, leaving low libido in the rearview mirror of your empowered journey.

Chapter 11:
Reigniting Passion

Reigniting passion starts with embracing both spontaneity and deliberate connection in your relationship. It's about rediscovering the thrill of intimacy and allowing yourself the freedom to explore what truly lights your fire. Sometimes, all it takes is a shift in perspective—transforming everyday routines into opportunities for romance, or reigniting flirtatious banter over a shared task. Trying new things can bring fresh energy; consider a weekend getaway or a daring new activity that brings out the adventurer in you both. The aim is to weave moments of intimacy into your daily life, to communicate desires and fantasies without fear, and to make space for a little mystery and allure. In this chapter, we'll explore both invigorating and soothing experiences, helping you and your partner become more attuned to each other's rhythms while fostering an environment where passion naturally flourishes.

Spice Up Your Love Life

Reigniting passion doesn't happen overnight, but it can start with small, intentional changes that add spice and excitement to your intimate life. Think of this journey not as a task list but as an opportunity to explore, define, and express what makes you and your partner feel alive and connected. This chapter isn't about transient sparks or temporary thrills. It's about cultivating enduring excitement and pleasure in your relationship, nurturing a space where your love continually grows and evolves.

Let's begin by exploring the idea of novelty. Our brains crave new experiences, and this desire for novelty is woven deeply into how we build and maintain passion. This doesn't mean you need to throw caution to the wind and become someone else entirely. It could be as simple as changing the setting. If you're used to keeping the bedroom door closed, perhaps it's time to let the outdoors in. A picnic in a secluded spot or a midnight gaze at the stars can set a romantic scene, and leads naturally into intimate connection.

Another way to introduce newness is through surprise. Small surprises, even in the form of a handwritten note or a thoughtful gift, can rekindle the excitement of early dating. These tokens communicate thoughtfulness and care, breaking the monotony that might have settled over time. Your aim is to bring back the attention and focus that often mark the early, passionate days of a relationship.

Communication, while crucial, becomes an evolving exchange of desires when aimed at adding spice to your love life. Start conversations around what you both imagine and desire, creating a safe space to express fantasies. These talks are not confinements; they are about opening doors. They allow both of you to share, discover, and try things that you might have been hesitant to explore. And remember, it's not about pressure to perform but about learning what truly brings joy and connection.

The art of teasing and anticipation can't be overstated. Flirting doesn't have to stop once you've been together for a while. Playful interactions throughout the day can build up anticipation for more intimate moments later. Whether it's through texts, glances, or touch, allowing that playful and teasing energy back into your life can revive the sparks that once flew uncontrollably.

Don't underestimate the power of exploring together. Whether it's a new hobby, a class, or simply an adventure, doing something new together can deepen your bonds and bring a fresh energy into your shared life. It's about seeing each other in different lights, in new scenarios, and recognizing the many dimensions of your partner, which often brings out new levels of attraction and desire.

Remember, foreplay doesn't have to begin in the bedroom. It can start at breakfast with a compliment, continue with a midday text that stokes desire, and slowly weave its way into your evening. Letting intimacy unfold throughout the day allows for a more relaxed, more naturally flowing connection when the time finally comes to be together. Explore fantasies not just as things to do but as stories you tell each other, narratives that bind your emotional and physical intimacy.

It's important to consider multiple forms of touch. Physical intimacy can vary greatly in its form and rhythm. Consider a gentle massage after a long day, warm and aromatic oils enhancing the sensations. Or imagine exploring new dance styles, where movement itself becomes a form of intimate expression, speaking in the language of the body.

Your environment plays a significant role, too. Think about the atmosphere you create. Changes could be as simple as lighting a scented candle or adding soft textures to your space. Senses are gateways to passion, and enriching them can transform even the most familiar surroundings into an enclave of emotion and desire. Ambiance is more than a backdrop; it's an invitation to leave the day behind and focus entirely on your shared moments.

Expand your repertoire by reading or watching something new together that deals with intimacy and relationships. These shared experiences can spark conversation and discovery. They can offer insights into each other's preferences and open discussions that might not have occurred otherwise.

Finally, remember the power of laughter in intimacy. A sense of humour can diffuse tension and strengthen bonds. Sharing a joke or a funny memory can remind you both of your fundamental connection, the friendship that underpins your romantic relationship. So don't be afraid to play, laugh, and let humour lighten the pressure and expectation surrounding your intimate life.

Your journey in spicing up your love life isn't just about adding sparkle; it's about deepening connection and authenticity. It's about learning to cherish every layer of your relationship, every moment of joy and togetherness, and using those as a foundation for a more fulfilling and exciting intimate life. Above all, it's about embracing your own desires and your partner's, crafting a relationship where both of you feel valued, understood, and irresistibly drawn to one another.

This endeavour is a testament to love's capacity to evolve and grow more profound over time. It affirms that no matter where you are in your journey, passion can always be revived, rediscovered, and reimagined, one intentional moment at a time.

Reconnecting with Your Partner

Reconnecting with your partner can be a profound journey of rediscovery. It's all too easy for the demands of daily life to erode the connection that once felt so natural and effortless. Yet, amidst the chaos, lies the potential to create a deeper, more meaningful bond. The key is to approach the task with an open heart, a willingness to learn, and a spirit of collaboration. After all, reigniting passion is not merely about physical intimacy; it's a dance of emotional synchrony and understanding.

The first step towards rekindling your relationship is genuine communication. Many couples find themselves sidelining honest dialogue in favour of routine exchanges. This accidental oversight can gradually weaken the intimate connection. To bridge this gap, take time to have uninterrupted conversations. Talk about things that excite you, not just chores or obligations. Share dreams, fears, and everything in between. When you openly share and listen to each other's narratives, you lay the groundwork for a deeper bond, fostering intimacy that stretches far beyond the bedroom.

Establishing these lines of communication often requires trust and vulnerability, both of which can be challenging to embrace. Acknowledge the small acts of intimacy that strengthen this trust. A gentle touch, eye contact that lets your partner know they're truly seen, or simply being present and attentive—these actions speak volumes. They may seem insignificant, but they cumulatively create a secure environment where emotional and physical connections can flourish.

Couples frequently underestimate the importance of time spent together without distraction. Setting aside technology and focusing solely on each other can be transformative. Consider going on a date without smartphones, taking a walk together, or cooking a meal as a team. Engaging in shared activities helps to reignite the mutual desires and interests that first brought you together. Remember, it's not always about what you do, but the intent and attention behind it.

Laughter and playfulness can be potent tools in restoring a sense of connection. Over time, relationships can become bogged down with seriousness and responsibility. Reintroducing light-heartedness and humour can unveil a forgotten side of your relationship. Create moments of joy by recalling amusing memories or trying new experiences together. This lightened atmosphere can significantly ease the path towards reigniting passion.

Physical intimacy, too, plays a vital role in reconnecting with your partner, though it may not be the starting point for everyone. Understandably, approaching this aspect can be daunting when faced with low libido. However, intimacy thrives on a foundation of trust and anticipating each other's needs. Take the time to explore and rediscover your bodies together, without the pressure of reaching a particular outcome. It's the journey of exploration that counts, allowing space for passion to flourish.

Moreover, understanding and respecting each other's sexual needs and boundaries is paramount. Discuss openly what feels enjoyable and what doesn't. Such conversations can seem difficult at first, but they pave the way for mutual growth. When partners support each other's sexual well-being and desires, they create a harmonious environment that's conducive to both personal and shared satisfaction.

Reconnecting with your partner also involves embracing change. People and relationships are dynamic, constantly evolving entities. Clinging to past patterns may hamper the potential for growth. Accept the changes in yourself, your partner, and your relationship. Approach the new with curiosity instead of resistance. This acceptance can rejuvenate your connection, allowing the passion to flow in unexpected and exciting ways.

Finally, cultivate gratitude within your relationship. Recognise and appreciate the efforts you both make, no matter how small they appear. Continuous appreciation can nurture love and intimacy, transforming every shared moment into an opportunity to strengthen your bond. Gratitude elevates the connection, making reinvigorating passion a shared goal rather than a personal struggle.

As you embark on the voyage of reconnecting with your partner, remember that it's a gradual and continuous process filled with learning and adaptation. Though challenges may arise, each step taken with understanding and commitment brings you closer to a richer, more passionate connection. Reigniting passion is not merely about reliving old flames; it's about embarking on a journey to create a new, brighter fire together.

Chapter 12:
Alternative Therapy Options

Embarking on the journey to rekindle your desire can be both exciting and daunting, but exploring alternative therapy options might just offer the transformative path you've been seeking. Complementary to traditional treatments, alternative therapies present a unique opportunity to delve into the holistic and deeply personal dimensions of sexual wellness. From sex therapy, which offers a safe space to navigate intimate challenges and bolster communication, to holistic approaches like acupuncture and aromatherapy that seek to harmonise body and mind, these therapies offer a refreshing perspective on desire. The key is to remain open to discovering what resonates with your individual needs. By embracing these innovative avenues, you're taking a proactive step towards empowering your sexual health, fostering a deeper connection with yourself, and reigniting the passion you deserve. As you venture into these alternatives, remember that you're not just enhancing your libido but nurturing a whole new way of relating to your body and desires.

Benefits of Sex Therapy

Sex therapy often remains an underestimated approach to addressing low libido. However, its benefits can be profound, offering a personalised and non-judgmental space for women to explore the intricacies of their sexual health. This therapeutic option empowers women to unlock suppressed desires and navigate the obstacles that might be contributing to low libido. By delving into the emotional, psychological, and relational components of one's sexual life, sex therapy helps in rediscovering the joy and vitality of intimacy.

One of the most significant benefits of sex therapy is the safe environment it provides. For many, discussions around sex can feel taboo or embarrassing, and having a professional help navigate these conversations can be liberating. In the therapy room, personal taboos and cultural barriers can be addressed candidly. This exposure often reveals that what one feels is neither uncommon nor insurmountable. The realisation that you are not alone can be a powerful motivator, relieving feelings of isolation and shame.

Beyond breaking down barriers, sex therapy focuses on the unique patterns and beliefs that could be affecting libido. Often, women may not be aware of the ingrained beliefs or past experiences shaping their current sexual attitudes and behaviours. A skilled therapist can guide the exploration of these deep-rooted issues, providing the opportunity to reframe perspectives and establish healthier relationships with one's sexuality. This process of understanding and restructuring often serves as a foundation for increased sexual desire and satisfaction.

Moreover, sex therapy can significantly enhance communication within a relationship. Many couples struggle with transparent and constructive dialogue about their sexual needs and desires. Therapy sessions provide structured ways to engage in these conversations, teaching skills that can be applied in everyday life. As partners learn to communicate more openly, new levels of intimacy and understanding emerge, positively impacting libido. The skills developed during therapy often transcend the sessions, fostering deeper connections and more fulfilling relationships.

For women dealing with anxiety or stress-related libido concerns, sex therapy offers targeted strategies to manage these factors. It's not uncommon for stress to act as a significant libido suppressor. Through therapy, women learn techniques to curb these anxieties, often through practices that involve mindfulness and stress reduction, essentially building a toolkit to handle pressures without sacrificing desire. This empowerment can renew interest in intimacy and foster a healthier landscape for sexual expression.

Sex therapy also respects the intersection of physical and emotional health. Many women combat physiological factors impacting libido, such as hormonal changes or medical conditions. While addressing sexual function, a sex therapist collaborates respectfully with other healthcare providers, offering an integrative approach that acknowledges the intersection of mind and body. This holistic view ensures that all aspects of a woman's health are considered, enhancing the efficacy of the therapeutic interventions.

In addition to therapy's intrinsic benefits, there's the motivational element of feeling heard and validated. For many, just knowing someone is actively listening and prioritising their sexual wellbeing can reignite a sense of self-worth and motivation to engage in their sexual lives more enthusiastically. Feeling understood and respected in therapy can become a cornerstone for building confidence, which naturally supports a vibrant sexual life.

For those in relationships, another pivotal benefit is the opportunity to work collaboratively with a partner. Joint sessions can redefine partnership expectations, fostering a supportive dynamic where each person's desires and boundaries are acknowledged and valued. The collaborative nature of sex therapy ensures that both members of a relationship are actively participating in cultivating a fulfilling sexual life, reducing feelings of burden or pressure on one partner.

Likewise, for women exploring their own bodies and desires independently, sex therapy might focus on self-exploration and understanding personal arousal patterns. Gaining insights into what specifically increases one's desire can lead to more self-assured interactions and a deeper connection to personal needs. This self-knowledge is invaluable, providing clarity that can boost libido through a stronger connection to one's body and mind.

Ultimately, the result of sex therapy transcends improved sexual experiences; it cultivates an empowered state of being where women can speak up for their desires with confidence. Women find themselves equipped with lifelong skills to not only manage libido fluctuations but to thrive in their sexual lives. This empowerment does not end with rekindled desire; it permeates all aspects of their lives, strengthening their voice in relationships and reinforcing their agency over their bodies.

In conclusion, the benefits of sex therapy are diverse and impactful. From fostering open communication to managing stress and redefining personal beliefs, it provides invaluable tools for women eager to reclaim their sexual vitality. Through a supportive therapeutic journey, women can experience not only a resurgence of desire but a profound transformation in their relationship with themselves and others. Embracing sex therapy is not just a step towards rekindled libido; it is a bold stride towards a more fulfilled and authentic life.

Exploring Holistic Approaches

In our journey through understanding and addressing low libido, it's essential to consider the value of holistic approaches. These methods acknowledge the intricate web of interactions between the mind, body, and spirit in shaping a woman's sexual well-being. By integrating these dimensions, holistic approaches offer an expansive view beyond just the physical symptoms, aiming to balance and harmonise aspects of life that contribute to sexual desire.

At its core, holistic health is about achieving balance. This notion recognises that low libido often stems from disruptions in mental or emotional well-being, physical health, and spiritual fulfilment. Unlike traditional methods focusing solely on physical causes, holistic approaches consider psychological aspects, lifestyle choices, and even the environment's impact on sexual health.

One popular holistic practice is the ancient tradition of acupuncture. This therapy, rooted in Traditional Chinese Medicine, involves inserting fine needles into specific points on the body to stimulate energy flow, or "qi". It's believed that acupuncture can help relieve stress, enhance circulation, and balance hormones, thus addressing some known factors contributing to low libido. Women have reported not only increased sexual desire but also a deeper sense of relaxation and clarity.

Herbal supplements also play a significant role in holistic health. Adaptogens such as maca root and ashwagandha are often used to support sexual vitality. These herbs can help the body manage stress and regulate hormones, providing a natural boost to libido. It's not just about the active compounds, but the ritual of self-care involved in selecting and using these supplements that fosters a sense of personal agency and empowerment.

Another aspect of holistic care is yoga and meditation. These practices encourage mindfulness, helping women connect with their bodies in a compassionate and non-judgmental way. Yoga, through its physical postures and breathing techniques, promotes relaxation, flexibility, and blood flow. Similarly, meditation offers a sanctuary for the mind, reducing stress and fostering a more profound sense of self-awareness.

The emotional benefits of yoga and meditation can't be understated; they provide a space to process emotions that might be hindering libido. By nurturing a peaceful state of mind, women can begin to unearth the roots of their inhibitions, fostering a healthier, more connected sense of desire. Over time, this practice can transform the way women relate to their bodies and their sexual selves.

Aromatherapy, often overlooked, can be another complementary tool in the holistic toolkit. Essential oils like ylang-ylang, sandalwood, and jasmine are renowned for their aphrodisiac qualities. By stimulating the limbic system, which is responsible for regulating emotions, these oils can subtly shift mood and arousal. Integrating aromatherapy into a daily routine, such as in baths or massages, can serve as a gentle reminder of sensuality and self-love.

Beyond these practices, the role of nutrition in holistic health can't be ignored. The foods we eat play a crucial part in maintaining hormonal balance and energy levels. A diet rich in whole foods, healthy fats, and antioxidants supports not just physical health, but mental clarity and mood. It's about creating a nourishing environment where libido can naturally flourish.

Incorporating holistic approaches isn't about replacing traditional treatments but rather complementing them. By embracing these methods, women can embark on a journey of self-discovery, where understanding personal rhythms and needs becomes a transformative experience. Every step towards integrating holistic practices can unveil new facets of sexuality, turning challenges into opportunities for growth.

Importantly, exploring holistic approaches invites women to think about their wellbeing as an interconnected system. It's a shift from a reactive to a proactive stance on health, where prevention and nurturing take centre stage. By empowering oneself with knowledge and practices that resonate personally, women can take control of their sexual health journey, fostering a sense of empowerment and self-advocacy.

As you explore these holistic avenues, consider what resonates with your unique experience. There's no one-size-fits-all, and that's the beauty of holistic health—it honours individuality and encourages exploration. Whether it's the calm of meditation, the energy of acupuncture, or the vibrant colours of a balanced meal, each choice is a step towards a deeper understanding of what your body needs to thrive.

This exploration isn't just about reclaiming a lost libido; it's about enriching one's entire life experience. A holistic approach promotes a more engaged, joyful existence where sexual desire is a natural, integrated part of a whole, healthy life. In this light, the journey to enhancing libido becomes an opportunity to live more fully and authentically.

Chapter 13:
Navigating Medical Treatments

Diving into the world of medical treatments for low libido can seem daunting, but understanding your options is a vital step towards rekindling desire and achieving a fulfilling sexual life. This journey often begins with recognising that hormonal therapies might offer relief, particularly for those experiencing shifts due to menopause or hormonal imbalances. Navigating these treatments requires careful consultation with healthcare professionals who specialise in women's sexual health, ensuring solutions are tailored to your unique needs. It's crucial to match medical interventions with informed conversations and an open mind, weighing potential benefits and side effects together. Remember, this path isn't just about leveraging treatments, but also about reclaiming control and empowering yourself through each decision, affirming your right to a satisfying sexual well-being. Embrace this exploration as part of a broader strategy that includes understanding and compassion for your body's needs, ensuring the most authentic path back to intimacy.

Understanding Hormonal Therapy

In the journey towards rejuvenating one's sexual desire, hormonal therapy emerges as a compelling, albeit sometimes complex, option. It's crucial to delve into this topic with an open mind and a willingness to navigate new information. Hormonal therapy isn't a one-size-fits-all solution; rather, it's a personalised approach that can significantly impact libido and overall well-being. Understanding its nuances can empower you to make informed decisions that align well with your desires and health goals.

At the heart of hormonal therapy is the idea of restoring balance. Hormonal changes, particularly those related to oestrogen, testosterone, and progesterone, can play a significant role in a woman's sexual health. These hormones are critical in maintaining various bodily functions, including mood regulation, energy levels, and most pertinently, sexual desire. A decrease in these hormones can lead to diminished libido, among other symptoms such as fatigue and mood swings. Hormonal therapy aims to replenish these hormones to their optimal levels, potentially rekindling the spark that once fuelled your passion.

Before diving headfirst into hormonal therapy, it's important to recognise that these treatments should be discussed extensively with healthcare professionals. Collaborating with an endocrinologist or a gynecologist can provide insights tailored to your unique needs. They can help determine if hormonal imbalances indeed contribute to low libido and discuss the risks and benefits of hormone replacement therapies—ranging from patches and pills to creams and injections.

It's worth noting that while hormonal therapy can positively impact libido, it may not be a magic bullet for everyone. The human body is an intricate web of interconnected systems, and libido is influenced by psychological, emotional, and relational factors alongside the physiological. This means that addressing low libido might require a holistic approach, combining hormonal therapy with other strategies discussed in this book, such as mindfulness, lifestyle changes, or even seeking relationship counselling.

Hormonal therapy often involves using bioidentical or synthetic hormones to either supplement or replace hormones your body is deficient in. Bioidentical hormones, created to chemically match the hormones produced naturally by the body, are frequently touted for their purported safety and efficacy. However, the debate on bioidentical versus synthetic hormones is ongoing, and research continues to evolve, underlining the need for informed decision-making.

Deciding to embark on hormonal therapy is a deeply personal choice, influenced by various factors including age, personal health, medical history, and personal preferences. Some women might seek it during menopause, where symptoms related to hormonal decline become more palpable. Others might explore this avenue post-hysterectomy or due to conditions like premature ovarian insufficiency.

Consider the practical aspects too. Hormonal treatments can vary greatly in administration methods, frequency, and potential side effects. Some women might experience relief and renewed energy quickly, while others might need dose adjustments to find their optimal balance. Common side effects could include bloating, weight changes, or mood swings, and it's vital to weigh these against the potential benefits.

Moreover, there are alternatives within the scope of hormonal therapy worth exploring. Selective Estrogen Receptor Modulators (SERMs) or Testosterone Therapy for women are also sometimes considered to enhance sexual function. Again, these should be discussed with a healthcare professional to understand their suitability and safety concerning your unique situation.

One can't ignore the profound impact that feeling in control of your sexual health can have on overall empowerment and confidence. Hormonal therapy presents an opportunity not only to address physical symptoms but also to take charge of your health narrative, reinforcing that your desire matters, and actively pursuing it is not only valid but crucial for a fulfilling life.

In conclusion, venturing into the realm of hormonal therapy requires a harmonious balance of knowledge, introspection, and professional guidance. It's about more than just correcting hormonal levels; it's about reawakening a part of yourself that may have felt dormant. Embrace the journey with curiosity and courage, knowing that tapping into your desires is not just vital to your sexual health but also integral to your overall sense of empowerment and well-being.

Other Medical Interventions

While hormonal therapy is a well-known approach to addressing low libido, there are various other medical interventions worth considering. Modern medicine offers a myriad of options that can aid in reigniting sexual desire. These solutions cater to different underlying causes of libido challenges, recognising that each woman's experience is unique. In exploring these interventions, a holistic view of your health is vital.

One of the promising routes in combating low libido is the use of medications specifically designed to enhance desire. Flibanserin, marketed as Addyi, is one such prescription drug. It works by targeting neurotransmitters in the brain, aiming to restore a balance that can enhance sexual desire in premenopausal women. It's important to consult a healthcare professional to understand the suitability and potential side effects of such medications.

In some cases, the use of antidepressants is implicated in reducing sexual desire due to their effect on neurotransmitters. This irony, given that these medications target mood disorders, highlights the complexity of the brain's chemistry. A medical professional might explore altering the dosage or trying different medications to mitigate such effects. It's a delicate balance but addressing it can make a significant difference in one's sexual health.

A lesser-discussed approach includes testosterone therapy, which is sometimes utilised off-label for women experiencing low libido, particularly post-menopause. Though traditionally seen as a male hormone, testosterone plays a crucial role in female sexual health as well. Research suggests that it can potentially enhance libido and sexual satisfaction. However, it's essential to approach this option with careful medical guidance, given the possible side effects and the controversial nature of its use in women.

Vaginal oestrogen treatments are another option for addressing sexual dysfunction, especially when symptoms like vaginal dryness accompany low libido. Oestrogen creams, tablets, or rings can be applied directly to the vaginal tissues, providing relief from discomfort during intercourse and aiding in restoring sexual desire. Localised treatments tend to have fewer systemic effects, making them a safe choice for many women.

Recent advancements have seen the emergence of laser therapies aimed at improving vaginal health. Although primarily used to address vaginal laxity and atrophy, these procedures can also enhance sexual enjoyment and reduce discomfort. By stimulating collagen production and improving vaginal elasticity, laser treatments might indirectly contribute to enhanced libido by making sexual activities more pleasurable.

Pelvic floor physical therapy can also serve as an effective intervention. As we age or undergo life changes like childbirth, the pelvic floor muscles can weaken, impacting sexual function. A pelvic floor therapist can tailor exercises to strengthen these muscles, potentially boosting sexual function and, subsequently, desire. Some women have reported heightened sexual pleasure as a result of strengthened pelvic floor muscles, making this an avenue worth exploring.

In certain cases, addressing underlying health issues can inadvertently improve libido. Conditions like diabetes, cardiovascular disease, or thyroid disorders can all play significant roles in reducing sexual desire. Managing these with appropriate medical interventions often results in a corresponding improvement in sexual health. Thus, a thorough health evaluation by a medical professional could be a critical step in the journey to reclaiming your libido.

Additionally, it's worth considering the impact of lifestyle medications, such as those for blood pressure or allergies, on sexual desire. Sometimes, the side effects of these medications can be the hidden culprits behind diminished libido. Discussing with your doctor the possibility of switching to alternatives with fewer sexual side effects might ease the issue.

Beyond pharmacological and physical interventions, psychological support remains a cornerstone in navigating medical treatments for low libido. Therapists specialising in sexual health can offer strategies and support to bolster confidence and interest in sexual activity. Cognitive behavioural therapy (CBT), for example, is beneficial in reframing negative thoughts about sex into more positive perspectives, thereby potentially reigniting interest and desire.

The key to navigating other medical interventions is collaboration with healthcare providers. By working closely with specialists, and being open about your concerns and experiences, you can craft a strategy that addresses your specific needs. Remember that informed decisions and proactive management are powerful tools in overcoming challenges.

Ultimately, these medical interventions provide a spectrum of options to suit different causes and manifestations of low libido. It's about finding what aligns with your personal health profile and lifestyle. By considering other medical interventions alongside lifestyle changes and emotional strategies, you can holistically approach the complex nature of sexual desire.

Chapter 14:
Self-Exploration and Masturbation

In the journey to rekindle your sexual desire, self-exploration and masturbation serve as empowering tools that foster a deeper understanding of your body and its responses. Engaging in this intimate practice not only enhances self-awareness but also nurtures a positive relationship with your sexuality, free from judgement or obligation. As you learn to embrace the nuances of your own pleasure, you gradually dismantle long-standing taboos, allowing space for curiosity and self-discovery. This personal exploration can lead to heightened arousal and confidence, paving the way for improved sexual interactions and deeper intimacy with your partner. By recognising and celebrating your unique pathways to pleasure, you're not just addressing low libido — you're building a more fulfilling sexual identity. Remember, this is a journey towards understanding and accepting yourself completely, freeing you to experience and express desire, unencumbered by external expectations.

Benefits of Self-Discovery

The journey of self-discovery is like peeling back the layers of an onion, each one offering new insights and revelations. When it comes to self-exploration and masturbation, this process does more than just foster a deeper understanding of your sexual self; it enriches numerous facets of your life. By embracing this exploration, women can embark on a transformative journey that reawakens their sensual potential, helping to navigate the path towards a more fulfilling sexual experience.

Firstly, self-discovery encourages a profound sense of autonomy and body confidence. Taking the time to explore one's own body without external pressure or expectations allows women to uncover what genuinely feels pleasurable. It's a powerful affirmation that their pleasure is both worthwhile and deserved. This autonomy isn't just about understanding the physical; it extends to emotional and mental realms. Feeling at home in one's skin provides the confidence to engage more authentically in intimate encounters, fostering a healthy self-image that naturally enhances libido.

Understanding personal arousal cues through self-exploration can also have significant benefits. Many women experience low libido due to a lack of connection with what truly turns them on. Masturbation acts as a form of practical education, allowing them to identify specific stimuli that ignite desire. This knowledge is crucial, as it creates a blueprint for communicating needs and preferences to partners, which is an integral step in creating mutually satisfying experiences.

The mental benefits of self-discovery run deep, particularly in overcoming societal pressures and misconceptions about female desire. Many women grow up in environments where discussions around self-pleasure are shrouded in taboo or downright discouraged. Embarking on this journey dispels such myths and normalises the conversation around female sexuality. It positions masturbation not as a solitary activity swathed in secrecy but as a healthy, empowering expression of self-love. By reclaiming this narrative, women dismantle shame and guilt, replacing them with self-acceptance and pride.

Moreover, self-exploration is a superb stress reliever, with the potential to address psychological factors affecting libido. In our fast-paced world, stress often acts as a significant barrier to sexual desire. Masturbation releases endorphins, the body's natural feel-good hormones, alleviating stress and fostering relaxation. This self-care activity offers a sanctuary from daily pressures, allowing women to reconnect with their bodies in a soothing and pleasurable way.

Interestingly, self-discovery also stimulates creativity and openness, transcending the boundaries of sexual experiences and impacting other life areas. Engaging with one's sensuality unlocks a flow state that can spark creativity. Some women find that this intimate exploration inspires them artistically or helps them think about challenges differently, nurturing an open mind that is as receptive to new ideas as it is to new sensations.

On a relational level, self-discovery enhances intimacy and connection with a partner. When women understand their bodies and desires, they are more equipped to create meaningful, intimate moments with others. This understanding and clarity foster ease and comfort in intimate settings, allowing for better communication, more joy, and deeper emotional bonds. Partners benefit from this knowledge, too, as it allows for building narratives around shared pleasure and lessens the fear of misunderstanding or rejection.

Masturbation as a tool for self-discovery also provides a testing ground for sensual experimentation. Without the pressure of performing for a partner, women can explore different techniques, fantasies, and toys, to discover what excites them. This no-pressure environment allows for valuable exploration, widening the potential for sexual experiences both alone and with a partner. It helps to keep the sense of curiosity alive, contributing to a dynamic and evolving sexual journey.

Additionally, self-exploration can play a crucial role in improving sexual satisfaction. Women who engage in regular self-pleasure develop an intimate knowledge of their bodies, which can lead to more satisfying and intense orgasms. Pleasure, like any skill, often benefits from practice and understanding, which is precisely what self-exploration provides. By demystifying one's own sexual responses, women can guide partners more effectively, leading to mutually gratifying experiences.

The process also nurtures mental health and emotional resilience, which are vital elements for combating low libido. By engaging with oneself in a caring and pleasurable way, women cultivate a mindset of nurturing and empowerment. This, in turn, fosters resilience, aiding in the management of life's myriad challenges. It reinforces the belief that women have the tools and power to satisfy their own needs emotionally, sexually, and otherwise.

Finally, the journey of self-discovery aligns beautifully with the broader ethos of empowerment and personal choice. In a world where women's bodies and desires have often been scrutinized and controlled, claiming ownership over one's pleasure is a radical act of self-advocacy. It's a message that their bodies belong to them and their choices about those bodies are valid and important. As women honour this path, they not only empower themselves but also contribute to changing the narrative for future generations who will perceive female desire as something natural, celebratory, and deeply personal.

Techniques for Personal Pleasure

Exploring the realm of personal pleasure can be a profoundly enriching experience. It's not just a physical journey but a voyage of self-awareness that allows you to understand your body in new and deeper ways. When you take the time to truly connect with yourself, you lay the foundation for a more fulfilling and satisfying sexual life. This process isn't merely about achieving climax, though that can be a delightful part of it. Instead, it's about cultivating a richer connection to your own desires and igniting a personal sense of empowerment.

To embark on this journey of self-discovery, begin by creating a space that feels both safe and inviting. An atmosphere that nurtures relaxation and free expression is crucial. This might involve tidying your bedroom, lighting a few softly scented candles, or playing your favourite tunes. Assess the lighting, temperature, and overall vibe of the room—perhaps there's a specific scent that helps you unwind. The goal here is to build an environment where you feel completely at ease.

Once you've cultivated a tranquil and welcoming atmosphere, attune yourself to the present moment. The practice of mindfulness can significantly enhance your experience, allowing you to focus entirely on the sensations and feelings your body communicates. Close your eyes, take deep breaths, and notice how your body feels. Stay present with each sensation, no matter how subtle it might be. This sort of mindful connection can increase your awareness, making the whole experience more pleasurable and insightful.

In the realm of techniques, there's a plethora you can explore, and each offers something unique. Consider starting with gentle caresses, experimenting with varying pressures and rhythms. Understand the geography of your body; learn what feels good and what brings little sparks of joy. Fingers are marvellous tools, but don't forget that exploring with other textures can introduce fascinating dynamics.

A key technique in cultivating personal pleasure involves understanding your breath. Breathwork isn't typically associated with sexual exploration, but it can profoundly impact your experience. Slow, deep breaths can heighten your sensations, while shallow, quick breaths can escalate excitement. Find a rhythm that aligns with your body's responses, and you might discover new dimensions to pleasure.

The choice of lubricant can also change the course of exploration. Natural oils such as coconut or almond oil provide a gentle glide, while a quality water-based lubricant might offer a slicker experience. Using a lubricant can eliminate unnecessary friction, allowing for a smoother, more comfortable exploration. Ensuring your choice is body-safe and compatible with both your skin and personal preferences is paramount.

Incorporating tools such as vibrating toys can add an exciting depth to self-exploration. The variations in rhythm and intensity provide new opportunities for discovering what specifically works for you. There's no rush; taking your time to experiment with different settings can enhance your understanding of your body's wants and responses. Remember, the key is curiosity rather than a goal-focused approach.

Beyond physical exploration, engaging your mind can intensify the experience of personal pleasure. Erotic literature or visual stimuli that resonate with you can unlock deeper layers of arousal, integrating imaginative elements with tangible ones. Let your mind wander freely to fantasies or scenarios that excite you, allowing desire to inform your exploration.

Furthermore, cultivating self-compassion is a fundamental aspect of this journey. Some may encounter moments of frustration or impatience, especially if climax feels elusive. It's critical to approach such feelings without judgment. Personal pleasure isn't about performance metrics but about embracing the joy of the experience itself. Practising patience and kindness with yourself is a powerful technique that can transform the journey entirely.

Self-exploration doesn't need to be a solitary or secret affair. Sharing your discoveries with a partner can open up avenues for enhanced intimacy. Communicating your insights allows both of you to appreciate and honour each other's desires more fully. Having discussions about what you've learned might even elevate shared experiences to new heights.

Ultimately, techniques for personal pleasure are deeply personal and can be as unique as the individuals exploring them. It's a continuous discovery, one that can shift and evolve over time. Embrace the changes, and let this journey be a source of empowerment and confidence. Understanding your pleasure is a step towards a more liberated and fulfilling sexuality, making this exploration an invaluable aspect of your personal growth.

Chapter 15:
Technology and Libido

In our ever-connected world, technology's role in shaping our desires is undeniable. While social media exposes us to idealised portrayals of love and intimacy, fostering unrealistic expectations that may dampen our genuine yearnings, it's crucial to remember it's a double-edged sword. On one hand, technology offers platforms to explore fantasies and communicate with partners in creative ways. On the other, it can lead to comparisons and distractions that hinder authentic connection. Pornography use, often viewed in secret, presents both opportunities for enhanced exploration and risks of desensitisation. It's about finding a personal balance—harnessing the benefits of technology to enrich, not replace, the human touch and communication we crave. By consciously navigating this digital landscape, you can better manage the noise and focus on nurturing a vibrant, intimate connection that aligns with your deepest desires and truest self.

The Impact of Social Media on Desire

In our hyper-connected world, social media has emerged as a powerful influence on various aspects of our lives, including our intimate expressions. For women grappling with low libido, understanding how this digital landscape impacts desire is crucial. Social media platforms aren't just communication tools—they're spaces where ideals and expectations are constantly curated and magnified, often in ways that can either inspire or undermine our sense of self.

Social media is a double-edged sword in the realm of intimacy and desire. On one hand, these platforms offer a wealth of information, connection, and community support, all of which can provide an empowering narrative around women's sexuality. On the other hand, they can also propagate unrealistic standards of beauty and performance, which, when internalised, may contribute to feelings of inadequacy or anxiety about one's sexual self.

Visual-centric platforms are particularly potent in shaping perceptions. The relentless display of 'filtered reality' can distort what is seen as normal, desirable, or attractive. Women may find themselves comparing their bodies, relationships, and sexual experiences to those idealised online portrayals. Over time, this comparison can lead to a decline in self-esteem and body confidence, both of which play significant roles in sexual desire.

Moreover, the curated life highlights seen on social media can create a sense of pressure to perform or achieve certain milestones in one's personal life. This subliminal pressure often creeps into the bedroom, leaving individuals feeling disconnected from their authentic selves. The consequence? A desire that gets suppressed under the weight of expectation and comparison.

However, all is not doom and gloom when it comes to the intersection of social media and libido. Empowering movements and communities thrive on these platforms, helping to redefine what sexual expression and desire look like. From body positivity influencers to communities promoting sexual health awareness, social media can be a nurturing environment that encourages exploration and acceptance.

Building a healthy relationship with social media requires mindfulness. Women can consciously curate their feeds to follow accounts that uplift rather than drain, substituting comparison for community. This positive digital ecosystem can serve as a supportive backdrop against which women can begin their journey of rediscovering desire.

It's crucial to recognise the transitory nature of trends and fads perpetuated online. What's fashionable might not be what is authentic or true for you personally. Embracing one's uniqueness in the face of homogenised ideals is a radical act of self-love that can liberate sexual desire from the constraints imposed by digital narratives.

Furthermore, setting boundaries with social media use is vital. Taking digital detoxes, engaging in offline hobbies, or practicing mindful use of technology can shift focus from screens to the tangible, fostering an environment where real desires can surface and be nurtured.

Social media also boasts an abundance of resources and knowledge sharing that can aid in demystifying sexual function and facilitate a deeper understanding of one's libido. Women can benefit from educational content, podcasts, and virtual discussions that equip them with insight and tools to enhance sexual wellness.

The impact of social media on desire underscores the importance of approaching online interactions with critical awareness. By leveraging the connectivity it offers while guarding against its pitfalls, women can reclaim their narratives and harness social media as a tool of empowerment rather than a harbinger of self-doubt.

In the grand tapestry of rediscovering libido, social media is just one thread. When wielded with intention and perspective, it can enhance the richness and depth of one's sexual identity—a testament to the intricate blend of technology and human emotion.

Navigating Pornography Use

Technology has undeniably woven itself into the fabric of our daily lives, influencing every aspect from work to leisure, and yes, even our sexuality. Pornography, once clandestine and tucked away in the dim corners of video stores, is now omnipresent, just a click away. While its pervasive presence can spark curiosity, it also poses complex challenges, particularly for women navigating low libido.

Understanding the intersection between pornography and personal desire is crucial. For some, pornography acts as a window into new fantasies, potentially spurring excitement and curiosity. It can serve as a tool for exploring one's sexuality in a private, consenting manner. However, for others, it may create unrealistic expectations and even feelings of inadequacy, impacting self-esteem and desire.

It's essential to approach pornography with a critical, mindful perspective. Ask yourself why you're drawn to it or how it makes you feel. Is it enhancing your sexual experiences, or is it creating a chasm between reality and expectation? For many women experiencing low libido, these are crucial questions that can lead to greater self-awareness and healing.

While pornography itself isn't inherently detrimental, it's the effects it can have on our perceptions of intimacy and self-worth that require scrutiny. Many studies point to the potential of pornography to shape unrealistic ideals of sexual interactions and body image. Engaging with these hyperbolic portrayals can sometimes distort our perception of what's normal or desirable, leaving some women feeling disconnected from their own bodies and desires.

The portrayal of women in pornography often reflects societal stereotypes, which can be damaging. These depictions can influence both partners' expectations about sex, further complicating matters when libido is already low. Communication and managing expectations become key factors in navigating these waters. Open discussions with partners about the consumption of pornography can be a stepping stone to rebuilding intimacy and establishing mutual understanding.

Technological advances have also led to the development of ethical and feminist pornography, which aims to portray more realistic, consensual, and diverse depictions of sex. For women looking to explore desires in a healthy way, seeking out these resources can be empowering. Such content might offer a positive contrast to mainstream material, allowing women to engage with erotica that aligns more closely with their values.

Self-compassion and patience are vital when navigating pornography use, particularly if you're grappling with low libido. It's okay to seek guidance and resources that can assist in evaluating how your consumption is impacting your sexual health. You're not alone in this journey, and recognising the need for adjustment is a step towards empowerment and improved wellbeing.

The goal isn't to banish pornography altogether but to harness its potential positively while being mindful of its limitations. Self-reflection can be a powerful tool in this process. Ask yourself how you feel during and after consuming pornographic content. Are there underlying emotions being stirred that need addressing? Self-awareness can lead to significant breakthroughs in understanding personal desires and rebuilding a connection with one's libido.

Another consideration is the impact of pornography on relationships. If partners have differing views about its usage or if it's causing tension, it's time to have an honest conversation. Navigating these discussions with transparency and empathy can clarify boundaries and lead to a healthier sexual relationship. Each partner's perspectives and feelings are valid, and finding common ground is essential for mutual respect and intimacy.

Reflect on how your use of technology, including pornography, affects your sexual habits. Do you find yourself spending more time with screens than with your partner? Prioritising real-life intimacy over digital consumption can help recalibrate your desires. Perhaps it's time to set boundaries on your technology use to foster a deeper connection with those around you and with yourself.

There's also the broader cultural context to consider—society often frames sex and desire through a very narrow lens, where pornography can serve as both a mirror and a magnifier. Challenging these narratives allows you to redefine what sexuality and desire mean for you personally. It's about reclaiming agency over your sexual health and not allowing external sources to dictate your experiences.

Ultimately, navigating pornography use is about finding what works for you individually and within your relationships. It's an opportunity to explore personal arousal with honesty and without judgment. Striving for balance, practicing mindful consumption, and establishing healthy boundaries are all part of a holistic approach to enhance your sexual wellbeing.

Visual media can be a complicated partner in the quest for libido liberation. Embrace the aspects that foster growth, exploration, and authentic connections while maintaining awareness of the potential pitfalls. Growth in understanding your own sexuality and the various influences on it can light the way back to desire, one informed choice at a time.

Chapter 16:
Overcoming Libido Challenges

In the journey to rediscover passion and desire, overcoming libido challenges often feels like navigating a complex maze, but it's not insurmountable. Understanding that persistent low libido can stem from a confluence of factors—psychological, physical, or relational— opens the door to targeted strategies that can help reignite your sexual vitality. It's crucial to approach these challenges with compassion, recognizing that some days will be more difficult than others. Integrating tailored strategies such as exploring new patterns of intimacy, adjusting lifestyle habits, or even seeking professional guidance can pave a constructive path forward. Remember, this isn't merely about reigniting desire; it's about embracing your sexuality with newfound confidence and forging a more fulfilling relationship with yourself and your partner. By acknowledging these challenges and actively pursuing solutions, you empower yourself to transform obstacles into opportunities for growth and deeper connection.

Strategies for Persistent Low Libido

As you're exploring this chapter, you might already recognise the importance of finding effective strategies for tackling persistent low libido. While women's sexual desires are multifaceted and definitely influenced by a myriad of factors, addressing the issue head-on can be transformative. The key is to approach it not as a daunting mountain to climb but as a journey of rediscovery. Sometimes, all it takes is a shift in perspective or a small change in routine to unlock a wealth of newfound desire.

Firstly, let's consider the power of reflection. Understanding where you are now involves looking back at what once sparked your desire. Reflect on times and experiences when you felt sexually alive and invigorated. What were the circumstances? Who were you with? What emotions were running through you? Taking the time to truly reflect can illuminate patterns or triggers that are impacting your current sexual health, providing insight into what strategies might work best for you moving forward.

Openly communicating with your partner plays a pivotal role. It's during these honest dialogues that you both can express desires and concerns, without judgement or defensiveness. Consider setting aside regular time for such discussions, treating them as an integral part of nurturing your relationship, much like date nights or shared hobbies. Remember, intimacy is not just about the physical—it's about emotional closeness and trust too.

Mindfulness, coupled with relaxation techniques, can do wonders for libido. Many women find that stress and anxiety are the silent saboteurs of their sexual desire. Harnessing mindfulness to reconnect with the present moment enables a more profound engagement with your senses, making intimacy more fulfilling. Techniques such as deep breathing, progressive muscle relaxation, or guided imagery can reduce stress responses, thereby clearing the mental clutter that often dampens libido.

Incorporating lifestyle changes, particularly in nutrition and exercise, can also be incredibly effective. While these may seem mundane in the context of improving libido, a balanced diet rich in libido-boosting nutrients and a consistent exercise routine can enhance overall energy levels, mood stability, and body image—all crucial components of sexual health. Simple swaps like integrating omega-rich foods or engaging in activities you genuinely enjoy, rather than simply exercising for the sake of exercising, can elevate both physical and emotional well-being.

Some women turn to holistic approaches, exploring options like acupuncture, yoga, or herbal supplements. While these are not one-size-fits-all solutions, they can complement other strategies. Practices such as yoga can synergise the mental and physical, promoting flexibility, circulation, and stress relief, which are all beneficial in reviving sexual interest.

Seeking professional support, such as sex therapy, can also prove invaluable. Engaging with a therapist provides a safe space to explore personal and relational factors contributing to low libido. They can tailor specific techniques to your individual experiences, equipping you with the tools to approach intimacy with confidence and curiosity.

Lastly, redefine and celebrate sensuality outside the traditional frames. This reformation could be as small as engaging in slow, mindful activities like bathing or dressing with intention, or gently exploring different forms of touch with your partner without expectations of intercourse. The aim is to kindle a deeper connection not only with your partner but with yourself.

In this ongoing journey, remember that persistence is key. Low libido might not vanish overnight, but with consistent application of these varied strategies, you're actively taking steps to enhance your sexual desire and, ultimately, your emotional and physical intimacy.

Coping with Libido Loss

When faced with the challenge of low libido, it can often feel like an uphill battle. You're not alone, and it's okay to acknowledge the frustration and confusion that might accompany this experience.

Coping with libido loss involves a multifaceted approach, addressing both the emotional and physical aspects of the issue. Understanding that your sexual desire is influenced by a complex interplay of factors is a crucial first step towards reclaiming it.

Let's start by recognising that libido is not a constant; it fluctuates with life events, relationship dynamics, and personal health. It's common for women to experience changes in their sexual desire as they age, enter different stages of life, or encounter stress. These fluctuations don't define you, and acknowledging them without judgment can provide a sense of relief.

One practical way to begin coping is through self-reflection. Take some time to consider any psychological factors that might be impacting your libido, such as stress, anxiety, or unresolved emotional issues. Journaling about these feelings or discussing them with a therapist may help unpack underlying concerns. It's not about finding quick fixes but rather fostering a deeper understanding of yourself.

Communicating openly with your partner about your experience is vital. It can prevent misunderstandings and build an environment of mutual support. Try sharing your feelings without placing blame, using "I" statements to express how you're feeling. For instance, "I've been feeling a bit disconnected lately and it's affecting my desire." Such conversations can lead to greater intimacy beyond the physical.

Physically, nurturing your body can have profound effects on sexual desire. Regular exercise, even in light forms like yoga or walking, promotes overall well-being and enhances body positivity. Similarly, paying attention to your nutrition can make a significant difference. Foods rich in vitamins, minerals, and antioxidants, such as fruits, vegetables, and whole grains, can support hormonal health, thus positively influencing libido.

As you cope with libido loss, consider introducing mindfulness practices into your routine. Mindfulness encourages you to be present in the moment, reducing stress and creating a connection with your body. Techniques such as deep breathing or meditation can be incredibly beneficial, fostering a calm mind and a relaxed body, which are conducive to an enhanced sexual experience.

It's also essential to explore your own body and understand what brings you pleasure. This journey of self-exploration can rekindle a sense of curiosity and fun in your sexual life, which in turn may boost your libido. Whether through self-touch or experimenting with different stimuli, becoming familiar with your likes and dislikes is empowering.

Addressing any psychological barriers through therapy can also offer a path forward. Cognitive-behavioral therapy, for example, is a structured approach that helps alter negative thought patterns that may influence your sexual desire. Seeking guidance from a professional can provide not only coping strategies but also validation and encouragement on your journey.

Don't underestimate the power of reconnecting with your sensuality through new experiences. Engaging in activities that bring joy or make you feel alive can indirectly benefit your libido. Attend a dance class, indulge in creative pursuits, or try activities that elevate your spirit. A fulfilled and joyful life outside the bedroom often translates into a richer sexual experience inside of it.

Finally, remember to cultivate patience. Coping with libido loss is a personal journey that takes time and introspection. It's important to honour your pace and give yourself permission to experiment, fail, and try again. Celebrating small victories along the way can maintain both motivation and optimism.

As you embark on the path to rekindling your desire, keep in mind that you're building a more intimate relationship with yourself and those you hold dear. Embrace this transformative process and acknowledge that seeking help when needed is a testament to your strength and commitment to your well-being.

Chapter 17:
Support Systems and Resources

In navigating the path to rediscovering your libido, the right support systems can be a catalyst for profound change. Reaching out for professional help, such as sex therapists or counsellors who specialise in sexual health, offers an opportunity for tailored guidance and understanding that's both reassuring and practical. These experts can illuminate the often tangled web of psychological and physiological factors influencing libido, helping to untangle them with empathy and expertise. Moreover, building a network of support amongst trusted friends or communities can provide a sense of belonging and understanding, reminding you that you are not alone in this journey. Engaging with support groups or online forums dedicated to women's health and sexuality can also be empowering, offering a safe space to share experiences, advice, and encouragement. Cultivating these connections not only fosters resilience but also inspires confidence as you take steps towards a more fulfilling and vibrant sexual life.

Finding Professional Help

Finding professional help can often be a transformative step in addressing low libido, particularly when navigating this complex issue feels overwhelming. Seeking guidance from a qualified professional offers not only expert insights but can also validate your experiences, making the journey toward rekindling desire less daunting. It's about giving yourself permission to seek the support that would best suit your unique needs.

Professional help can take many forms, yet identifying the right kind of support is crucial. One should start by considering a sexual health specialist or therapist. These professionals are trained to understand the multifaceted nature of libido and can provide tailored recommendations, helping you uncover underlying causes that might not be immediately apparent. Whether the issues stem from psychological factors, such as anxiety or depression, or are more rooted in physical health concerns, an expert's guidance can be invaluable.

It's important to acknowledge that feeling hesitant about discussing such intimate matters is completely normal. Many women find it challenging to open up about issues related to sexual desire, often due to embarrassment or shame. Yet, mental health professionals and therapists in this field are skilled at creating a safe and non-judgmental space for you to express your concerns. Their role is not to judge but to listen and provide thoughtful insights and strategies that align with your personal goals.

Consider, for instance, engaging with a sex therapist. Sex therapy can be incredibly empowering, offering a platform for understanding how your past experiences, emotions, and relationships influence your current libido. It's not merely about addressing the physical aspects of desire but delving deeper into emotional and relational contexts. Sex therapists guide you through this exploration with sensitivity, equipping you with tools to enhance intimacy and pleasure.

In addition to individual therapy, couple's therapy is a worthwhile consideration for those who perceive that their partnership dynamics contribute to their low libido. Therapists specializing in this area can assist both partners in communicating effectively about their sexual needs and desires, potentially healing any rifts and fostering a more supportive environment. Exploring these dynamics with a professional can cultivate greater empathy and understanding, which are vital components of a thriving sexual relationship.

Moreover, consulting with a healthcare professional, such as a GP or a specialist in women's health, can provide insights into any potential physiological factors involved. Hormonal imbalances, side effects of medications, or underlying health conditions might contribute to low libido, and addressing these with medical intervention can be critical. Having an open conversation with your doctor about symptoms and concerns can facilitate a better understanding of any medical treatments or lifestyle adjustments that might aid in regaining libido.

For many women, integrating holistic or complementary therapies alongside professional health services can also be beneficial. Practices such as acupuncture, yoga, and mindfulness are often used to enhance overall wellbeing and can have positive effects on sexual health. Consulting with practitioners who specialise in these areas can help you to explore options that might work harmoniously with traditional treatment approaches, providing a comprehensive toolkit for impacting your libido positively.

Navigating the healthcare system and finding the right professional can seem daunting at first, particularly when it feels like there are multiple avenues to pursue. It's often helpful to start by researching credentials and specialities, or seek recommendations from trusted friends or family members who might have embarked on similar journeys. Remember that this process is not a one-size-fits-all — it's about finding the professional help that feels aligned with your unique situation and comfort level.

Another crucial aspect is considering your comfort concerning cultural competency and inclusivity. It's vital to ensure that the professionals you consult respect your values, beliefs, and identity, fostering an environment where you feel respected and understood.

This alignment can significantly impact the effectiveness of the help you receive, ultimately contributing to a more positive outcome.

Cost is another factor to bear in mind, though it's important not to let financial concerns deter you from seeking essential support. Many professionals offer sliding scales based on income, and some community health services provide affordable counselling options. Additionally, some therapy might be covered by health insurance, so checking with your provider can help clarify what might be included.

In summary, finding professional help is about enhancing your journey with expertise and empathy. It's critical to recognise that seeking help is a strength, not a weakness, and choosing to work with a professional underscores your commitment to your wellbeing and sexual empowerment. Ultimately, the guidance and support offered by professionals can pave the way for rediscovering your libido and fostering deeper connections with yourself and your partner. This step, though at times intimidating, can unlock pathways to a more fulfilling and enjoyable sexual life.

Building a Supportive Network

Navigating the journey to reclaiming one's libido can sometimes feel like an uphill shift filled with moments of uncertainty and introspection. During these times, having a supportive network becomes an invaluable resource, something that can make all the difference. It's not just about leaning on those close to you but actively building a coalition of allies who uplift and empower you. Forming connections with others who can empathise with your experiences brings a sense of solidarity, which is crucial for emotional well-being.

In today's world, where everyone seems perpetually busy, building a supportive network might seem daunting. However, it's essential to recognise that support can manifest in many forms. It doesn't always have to be face-to-face interactions; virtual connections also count.

Technology offers a plethora of platforms to connect with communities and individuals who share similar experiences and goals. Social media groups, online forums, and dedicated websites can be wonderful venues for finding such support.

Think of friends and family as the cornerstone of this network. Often, your closest companions can provide understanding and a listening ear. Sharing your journey with them might feel vulnerable at first, but doing so can cultivate deeper intimacy and empathy. It's crucial to communicate your needs and what kind of support you're looking for, whether it's a chat over coffee or a shoulder to lean on during challenging periods.

Besides friends and family, consider seeking out support groups specifically focussed on issues surrounding female libido and sexual health. Many find solace and empowerment in groups where there's no judgement, only shared experiences and mutual encouragement. Such groups allow you to explore and express your feelings in a safe environment, providing insights into how others have navigated their unique journeys.

Sometimes, the challenges you face might require professional guidance. Building connections with healthcare professionals, therapists, or sex educators can offer expert perspectives and strategies you might not have considered. These professionals can be your allies, guiding you towards your goals with empathy and understanding rooted in expertise. They can also help normalise your experiences, which can be reassuring when facing struggles with libido.

Don't underestimate the power of mentorship. While it might not be the first thing that comes to mind in this context, finding a mentor who either professionally or personally understands your journey can be incredibly impactful. They can offer insights and advice from their own experiences, providing valuable guidance as you work through your challenges. A mentor could be someone you've met through a workshop, seminar, or even a mutual connection.

Within your circle, it's also beneficial to foster mutual support. Often, focusing on amplifying the voices and experiences of others within your network can create a ripple effect, encouraging open dialogue and shared empowerment. Celebrating each other's victories, no matter how small, and offering emotional support can build a cohesive community where everyone thrives.

Remember, it's important to establish boundaries even within supportive networks. Sometimes well-meaning advice can come across as overwhelming or not applicable to your situation. It's perfectly acceptable to politely decline suggestions that don't align with your needs. Communicating your comfort levels and boundaries helps maintain the integrity of your network, ensuring it remains a source of positivity rather than stress.

Strive to approach this journey with openness and gratitude. Recognise and appreciate the unique contributions of each member of your network, and express thankfulness. When the people in your network see their impact, it cultivates a spirit of giving that reinforces the community. This collective empowerment nurtures resilience, making the journey to rediscovering your desires not just easier but more enriching.

Ultimately, building a supportive network is about creating a compassionate ecosystem—one where you are both supported and supportive. It's a reciprocal relationship that can offer comfort, broaden perspectives, and empower you to take bold steps towards reclaiming your libido. While this is ultimately a personal journey, knowing you have a solid foundation of support can indeed make it feel less solitary and more of a shared adventure.

Chapter 18:
Communicating Needs and Desires

Opening the door to honest communication about your needs and desires can often feel daunting, yet it's a vital step toward reinvigorating a fulfilling sexual connection. Speaking up doesn't just invite understanding; it strengthens the bond, nurturing intimacy that goes beyond words. This chapter focuses on transforming silence into shared dialogue, empowering you to articulate what's truly important in your intimate life without fear or hesitation. It's about acknowledging your desires as valid and worthy, encouraging you to be bold in expressing them with openness and clarity. By fostering an environment where both partners feel heard, valued, and respected, you're laying the groundwork for a deeper emotional and physical connection. Remember, every relationship thrives on genuine communication, so let's dismantle the barriers that hinder it and embrace the power of being vulnerable and authentic with your partner.

Tips for Open Dialogue

Starting a conversation about intimacy and sexual desires with your partner can be daunting. Many people worry about vulnerability, misunderstandings, or the possibility of being judged. Yet, the benefits of open dialogue are immense, fostering deeper connections and mutual understanding. To communicate effectively about such sensitive matters, it's important to create a safe environment where both you and your partner feel comfortable expressing yourselves. This can be the foundation for nurturing a healthy sexual relationship.

Begin by choosing the right moment. Timing can make all the difference when opening up such conversations. Opt for a moment when neither of you is stressed or preoccupied; for instance, after sharing a meal or spending a relaxed evening together. The setting should be private and distraction-free, ensuring both of you can listen and be heard without interruptions. Ensure that you're both mentally and emotionally prepared for an honest conversation.

When discussing your needs and desires, clear and gentle communication is key. It's helpful to use "I" statements that express how you feel, which can prevent your partner from feeling accused or defensive. For example, instead of saying, "You never touch me anymore," try, "I feel more connected when we touch, and I'd like to experience that more often." This approach focuses on your experience and can guide the conversation toward constructive outcomes.

Moreover, active listening is crucial in maintaining open dialogue. Encourage your partner to share their thoughts and concerns, and truly listen without interruption. Show empathy for their perspective and validate their feelings, even if they differ from your own. You might say, "I can understand why you feel that way," or "Your feelings are important to me, and I want to understand." Such affirmations demonstrate that you care and are invested in your partner's emotional experience.

It's also important to manage expectations and be flexible. Conversations about intimacy can sometimes reveal differences in desires or misunderstandings. Approach these revelations with an open mind, and be willing to compromise where needed. Establishing mutual goals and exploring solutions together can be empowering.

This not only helps in navigating the intricate dynamics of desire but also strengthens the bond between you both.

Humour, when used appropriately, can also be a valuable tool in conversations about intimacy. Light-heartedness can ease tension and make discussions feel less heavy or confronting. Laughing together can reinforce your connection and help you both feel more at ease in tackling complex issues. However, ensure that humour is in sync with your partner's comfort level and doesn't downplay serious feelings or concerns.

In some cases, differences in communication styles can act as barriers. If one partner prefers direct conversations and the other is more reserved, finding a middle ground is key to effective dialogue. This might mean setting aside regular times to talk or using written communication if face-to-face talks feel too intimidating. Being mindful of each other's communication preferences respects individual differences and lays the groundwork for a more successful conversation.

Trust is fundamental in any dialogue about intimate desires. Without trust, sharing personal experiences and needs can lead to vulnerability or misinterpretation. It's essential to reassure your partner that their confidence is held sacred and that you're a team facing challenges together. Trust grows from consistent, respectful communication over time. By honouring this trust, you create a space where authentic and meaningful conversations thrive.

Practice patience and persistence. Not every conversation will resolve all issues or meet all needs instantly. Sexual desire and relationships are dynamic, evolving aspects of life. Regularly revisiting conversations about intimacy ensures that issues are addressed, changes are acknowledged, and both partners are on the same path. View it as an ongoing journey rather than one-time discussions.

Lastly, consider seeking external guidance if necessary. Professionals, like sex therapists or couple's counsellors, offer invaluable insights and can facilitate discussions in a supportive environment. They can provide tools and strategies to improve communication and resolve concerns. Inviting a neutral third party may alleviate pressure and progress the conversation in healthy, constructive directions.

In sum, open dialogue about needs and desires isn't just about managing low libido; it's a gateway to enhanced intimacy and understanding. As you navigate these conversations with care, compassion, and collaboration, your relationship's strength and satisfaction can blossom and endure.

Understanding and Expressing Your Needs

Understanding and expressing your needs is an essential step towards nurturing a fulfilling sexual life. It requires self-awareness and a willingness to explore your personal desires, emotions, and boundaries. Many women who experience low libido often feel disconnected from their sexual selves, leading to frustration and confusion. Recognising this is the first step in a journey towards reconnection and empowerment.

The foundation of expressing your needs lies in understanding them yourself. This involves delving deep into your own psyche and identifying what you truly desire. It's about acknowledging any misconceptions or societal pressures that may have clouded your self-perception. Think about how past experiences, beliefs, and cultural teachings have influenced your current understanding of your own needs. It's crucial to separate these external influences from your authentic desires.

Spend time reflecting on what sparks your interest, even outside the bedroom. What captivates your senses? Are there moments when you feel most alive? These reflections can provide clues to your true desires. Don't hesitate to write them down or discuss them with a trusted friend or therapist. This process can feel daunting at first, but it is necessary to break free from any inhibitions and fully embrace your sexuality.

Once you begin to gain clarity on your needs, the next step is to express them. Communication is vital for fostering intimacy and connection with your partner. Attempting to have these conversations might feel awkward initially, especially if discussing intimate matters isn't common in your relationship. Start by choosing a comfortable setting where you both feel relaxed and open.

While expressing your needs, it's important to communicate from a place of vulnerability rather than expectation. Use "I" statements to convey your feelings and desires. For example, say, "I feel close to you when we spend time touching each other," rather than, "You never touch me anymore." This method fosters a non-defensive environment where both partners feel safe to share and listen.

Be prepared to encounter some challenges during these conversations. There might be moments when emotions run high, or disagreements arise. It's crucial to remain patient and empathetic, both with your partner and yourself. Understand that miscommunications can occur, and that's perfectly normal. The goal is not to have a perfect conversation but to make progress in understanding each other's perspectives and needs.

If at any point it feels too overwhelming to navigate this alone, consider seeking support from a therapist who specialises in sexual health. They can provide guidance and techniques to improve communication and understanding between partners, ultimately helping you express your needs more effectively.

Learning to understand and express your needs also extends beyond verbal communication. Pay attention to non-verbal cues like body language and physical touch. Often, these gestures can convey desires and emotions as powerfully as words. Touch can have an immensely grounding effect, enhancing your connection with your partner and your own body. Exploring these dynamics can reveal much about your unspoken needs and preferences.

Remember, the journey of understanding and expressing your needs is deeply personal. It involves unlearning societal norms that may have conditioned you to suppress your desires. Embrace this journey as a path to empowerment, acknowledging that your needs are valid and deserve to be heard. By fully understanding and expressing what you want, you empower yourself to pursue intimacy and pleasure on your own terms.

Ultimately, this process isn't just about improving sexual desire; it's about enriching your entire life. Your needs and desires are reflective of your broader emotional and psychological health. Addressing them actively enhances not just your relationship, but your overall sense of self. It can lead to a more authentic, connected, and vibrant existence, both inside and outside the bedroom. Enjoy this newfound understanding as it guides you towards a more fulfilling sexual and personal life.

Chapter 19:
Creating a Sex-Positive Environment

In the journey to rediscovering desire, creating a sex-positive environment acts as a powerful catalyst. It involves transforming not just our physical surroundings but also the mental and emotional spaces we inhabit. The ambience of your home can be a direct reflection of how you perceive and embrace your sexuality. Start by infusing your environment with elements that promote relaxation and openness; this might include ambient lighting, soothing music, or personal touches that make you feel grounded and connected. Open and honest conversations are equally vital—encourage dialogues that break down taboos and foster understanding, both with yourself and your partner. By actively choosing to surround yourself with positivity and acceptance, you lay the groundwork for a nurturing and encouraging atmosphere that supports your sexual well-being. Embrace this space as a sanctuary where judgement is absent, inviting comfort and authenticity that ultimately empowers you to feel more in control and confident in your sexual expression.

Cultivating Positivity in Your Space

Crafting a sanctuary that invites and nurtures positivity is pivotal in creating a sex-positive environment. Your physical surroundings influence your psychological state more than you might realise. A space that's charged with negative energy or clutter can become a metaphorical barrier between you and your desire. As you embark on the journey to rekindle your libido, creating a welcoming, positive space could be one of the most profound steps you take.

Imagine entering a room that's dimly lit with soft, warm lights. The air is fresh, perhaps scented lightly with a fragrance that stirs something within you—maybe it's the subtle hint of lavender, or the sweet, earthy undertones of sandalwood. The textures around you are inviting—soft cushions, a cosy throw, smooth sheets. This isn't just a room; it's a haven, a place where you can escape from the stresses of the outside world and reconnect with yourself. Everything in this space encourages you to be present, to be mindful, and to be open to whatever comes.

Creating this kind of space doesn't require a dramatic overhaul of your living environment or excessive expense. Start with small changes that resonate with you. Consider the lighting: natural light can invigorate, whereas soft, ambient lighting can relax. Perhaps you'll find that a new throw pillow or a tactile blanket makes your bedroom feel more inviting. Consider also the colour palette—calming hues like blues or greens can create a soothing atmosphere, while warmer shades might energise and enliven you.

Beyond the aesthetic, it's essential to consider the practical. A cluttered room often reflects a cluttered mind. There's merit in decluttering not only for physical appeal but for mental clarity. Start with simple steps, maybe dedicating ten minutes each day to clearing a specific area. The act of decluttering can itself be meditative, allowing you to shed not only physical items but psychological burdens as well.

This space, however, is not solely defined by physical objects. It's also about what you allow into your mind and life. Cultivating positivity means being selective about the media you consume, the voices you amplify, and the energies you let into your space. Take a moment to consider the emotional weight of the books on your bedside, the playlists you listen to in this room, or the social media accounts you follow from here. Consider whether they uplift and empower you or add to the stress and negativity that can hamper sexual desire.

Another important aspect of cultivating positivity in your space is infusing it with personal meaning. This could mean displaying photos or mementoes that remind you of happy moments or aspirations. You might incorporate elements that connect you to your body and sensuality—whether it's silky sheets that feel luxurious against your skin or art that inspires and captivates you. Personal touches can shift a space from merely functional to deeply therapeutic.

But even the most emotionally and aesthetically perfect space can't cultivate positivity if it feels foreign or contrived. Authenticity is important, and your environment should reflect who you are and who you wish to become on this journey. Perhaps plants invigorate you, symbolising growth and renewal. Or maybe a serene, minimalist setup appeals, embodying relaxation and simplicity. Your preferences are key to creating a space that's truly personal.

Moreover, it's important to remember that this process is not about striving for perfection but about creating a setting where you feel comfortable and empowered. It's about fostering a connection with your space that'll support you in exploring and understanding your libido. If something doesn't feel right, be willing to make adjustments. Listen to what gives you joy, what relaxes you, and respond to it.

Once your space is physically prepared, use it to engage in practices that promote positivity and sexual energy. This could involve mindfulness exercises, yoga, or even dancing when no one is watching. Utilising your environment as a safe space for exploration allows you to engage with your desires without judgement or expectation.

Ultimately, the goal is to create a space that not only feels safe and inviting but also breathes positivity into your journey towards a more fulfilling sexual life. When your environment is in alignment with your inner intentions, it becomes a potent ally in your endeavour to rekindle desire.

If you've ever stepped into a place that felt inherently right—as if it was speaking to some part of you—you know the importance of cultivating the right energy. By shaping your physical surroundings to be a positive and inviting space, you're nurturing yourself in a way that encourages openness, self-exploration, and ultimately, sexual wellness.

Encouraging Open Conversations

Talking openly about sex is often easier said than done, even in intimate relationships sharing a home and life together. Many women grapple with cultural taboos and internal hesitations when it comes to articulating their desires and needs. Yet, open conversations are essential for creating a sex-positive environment where understanding, growth, and intimacy can flourish. Bringing these discussions into our lives can allow for deeper connections with both ourselves and our partners.

In this journey towards open communication, identifying hurdles is a crucial step. Fear of judgement or rejection often sits at the heart of these hurdles. Many women worry about how they may be perceived, fearing vulnerability could lead to diminished intimacy. But, it's important to remember that discussing our desires openly can foster greater intimacy rather than weaken it. It allows both you and your partner to align on expectations, discover mutual interests, and address potential conflicts preemptively.

Cultivating a space for these conversations takes deliberate effort. It's about setting an emotional and physical environment where both parties feel safe to express their thoughts without fear. This could mean scheduling a specific time to talk, ensuring that no interruptions occur, and both partners entering the discussion with an open mind and readiness to listen. It's about turning towards each other with curiosity rather than turning away with criticism.

The language we use during these conversations is vital too. Speaking clearly but compassionately can make a world of difference. Use "I" statements to express feelings—such as "I feel" or "I need"—to avoid placing blame or causing defensiveness. This way, discussions become less about pointing fingers and more about mutual understanding. For instance, instead of "You never make time for us," try "I feel a deep need for more together time with you."

Beyond verbal communication, let's not forget non-verbal cues. Body language mirrors emotions and intentions, often revealing more than words themselves. A soft touch, maintaining eye contact, and maintaining an inviting posture can communicate compassion and openness. When discussions escalate, a reassuring gesture can bring the conversation back to a more constructive path.

Encouraging open conversations also involves a commitment to being an active listener. Listening actively is more than just hearing words; it's about understanding and processing what's being communicated. It means being present and showing empathy by acknowledging feelings and asking clarifying questions when needed. When your partner speaks, nod to show understanding or restate what you've heard to confirm that the message received is correct.

Let's remember that open conversations are not solely about verbal exchanges. Sometimes silence speaks volumes too. Allowing moments of silence gives each participant time to think and process emotions. It's perfectly okay to pause when conversations become intense, giving the other party the opportunity to reflect on what's being discussed.

Resilience is a quality you may find invaluable on this journey. Not all conversations will proceed smoothly. Some attempts will be more difficult than others, especially when encountering sensitive or triggering topics. What's important is to remain persistent and compassionate, even if progress comes slowly. Applauding small victories can sustain motivation; each honest expression and respectful reception is a step towards a healthier sexual dynamic.

Introducing playfulness into conversations can ease tensions around challenging topics. Playfulness doesn't undermine the seriousness of the conversation but introduces lightness that can encourage openness. Laughing together can dispel discomfort, reminding both parties that they're in it together. Sharing intimate goofs or fantasies can also be a fun way to bond and discover new aspects of each other's desires.

Furthermore, encouraging open conversations shouldn't be limited to partners alone. Speaking with friends in supportive environments can offer fresh perspectives and reduce feelings of isolation often associated with low libido. Insightful exchanges with those who've faced similar challenges can provide comfort, lend strategies, and validate personal experiences in ways that partners may not be able to.

For those who find it exceptionally challenging to broach these conversations, professional guidance might offer a helping hand. Therapists and sexologists are trained to facilitate dialogue in a safe, structured setting. They can offer both strategic approaches and neutral perspectives that guide toward solutions. Often, professional environments provide the right mix of distance and expertise to help navigate tricky conversations.

In our pursuit of a sex-positive environment, it's crucial to remain open to evolving discussions. As we grow, so will our desires and understanding of them. Revisiting these open conversations, both with ourselves and our partners, ensures that everyone remains aligned, allowing room for changes in desire and new discoveries. It's a lifelong dialogue that feeds into greater intimacy and personal empowerment.

Ultimately, it's about empowering yourself to speak from the heart. Embrace vulnerability as a strength, allowing yourself to be seen, heard, and understood. It's in these genuine moments of connection that intimacy thrives, and a deeper appreciation for one another is cultivated. Conversations about sex aren't just about overcoming low libido—they're an integral part of weaving a rich tapestry of experience, support, and desire into your life.

Chapter 20:
Empowerment and Self-Advocacy

Empowerment in your sexual health journey begins with recognising your unique desires and taking ownership of your well-being. As you navigate the complexities of libido, it's crucial to embrace self-advocacy, transforming knowledge into action that aligns with your personal values and needs. Start by setting boundaries and communicating desires with confidence and clarity, ensuring your voice is heard in any relationship. Delve into the exploration of your body and mind, understanding that empowerment is not a destination but a continuous process of self-discovery and growth. Celebrate small victories, knowing each step taken towards self-advocacy leads to enriched and fulfilling sexual experiences. Let yourself be guided by intuition, supported by informed choices, and inspired by the freedom to craft the narrative of your desire on your own terms.

Taking Charge of Your Sexual Health

Stepping into the driver's seat of your sexual health journey is an empowering act. It challenges societal norms and recognises your needs as paramount. As you embrace self-advocacy, you'll discover your unique path to sexual wellness, transforming challenges into opportunities for growth. Assessing your sexual health isn't just about solving problems; it's a celebration of your sexuality as a vital aspect of who you are. After all, understanding your libido is just as much about nurturing your essence as it is about enhancing your relationships.

Your sexual health plays a significant role in your overall well-being. Low libido may sometimes nudge you towards deeper self-reflection, prompting questions about lifestyle, mental health, or relationships. Instead of shying away from these reflections, embrace them as a chance to explore what truly brings you joy and satisfaction. Taking charge means listening closely to both your desires and discomforts and recognising the narratives around sexuality that have influenced you.

The first step in reclaiming your sexual health involves education and awareness. Understanding how your body responds and what it needs, in terms of emotional, mental, and physical support, creates a foundation of knowledge that can guide you toward informed decisions. Explore how elements like hormones, stress, and nutrition intersect with your libido, as knowledge equips you to make empowered choices about your body and desire.

Diversity in resources is another key component of self-advocacy. The path to understanding and revitalising your libido isn't a narrow alley with one destination. It's more akin to a vibrant garden, offering varied sources of support—from professional guidance in therapy to community discussions and self-help readings. By seeking diverse perspectives, you enhance your capacity to advocate for your unique needs.

Interacting with health professionals with confidence and asserting your sexual health needs is a potent form of self-advocacy. Prepare for appointments by understanding the questions you have about your libido, and don't hesitate to bring up concerns, no matter how trivial they might seem. The relationship with your health practitioner should be a collaborative partnership focused on your goals.

It's also important to engage with your partner, should you have one, as part of this journey. Facilitating open, sincere discussions about libido challenges and desires not only improves mutual understanding but also fosters a supportive environment where both partners feel heard and validated. This discourse can build intimacy and trust, pivotal in navigating the ebbs and flows of sexual desire together.

Don't overlook the power of personal introspection. Journaling about your feelings related to sexual desire, reflecting on past experiences, and regularly checking in with yourself to identify shifts in your mental and physical states can reveal underlying patterns. Self-reflection becomes a tool for identifying what changes, if any, need to be made and what aspects are worth exploring further.

Embracing flexibility in your approach is essential. As you navigate through different strategies, be gentle with yourself. Some discoveries may resonate deeply, while others may not bring the expected results. The key lies in maintaining an open, curious mindset, where each experience is part of the broader journey, not an end in itself.

Your sexual health empowerment doesn't stand in isolation. Consider your broader support network. Engage with communities that advocate for similar quests, whether online forums, book clubs discussing sexual wellness literature, or local health workshops. Interacting with a community that shares and supports your journey can offer additional insights, compassion, and even friendship.

It's vital to recognise that empowerment isn't a destination—it's a continuous journey filled with learning, growth, and self-discovery. As you create a supportive, liberating environment for your sexual health, encourage a mindset of ongoing curiosity and adaptability.

In the landscape of sexual health, self-care forms another cornerstone of empowerment. This encompasses everything from ensuring adequate rest and relaxation to engaging in activities that make you feel radiant and alive. Actions like practising mindfulness, focusing on mental health wellness, and cultivating an active lifestyle all reinforce your commitment to self-care.

Remember, empowering your sexual health is about taking practical steps. Set goals that align with your needs and values. Whether it's adopting new habits, seeking therapy, or reading up on ways to enhance libido, these practical steps are evidence of your commitment to your well-being.

Ultimately, taking charge of your sexual health is about reclaiming your narrative. It's about understanding that your desire is worthy of attention and care. As you advance in your journey, you're not just seeking to reignite libido but also to celebrate and nurture a vital part of yourself—unabashed and confident, living a life attuned to your desires and well-being.

Empowering Personal Choices

When it comes to sexual desire, empowerment and self-advocacy are indispensable allies. They're the tools that allow you to take charge of your sexual health and make choices that align with your personal values and desires. It's about crafting a sexual narrative that's authentically yours, free from societal expectations or stereotypes. This section is dedicated to exploring the myriad of ways in which personal choices can be empowered, arming you with the agency needed to shape your intimate life as you see fit.

Understanding your own needs is the cornerstone of empowering personal choices. Knowing what you want—or discovering it—is a journey that's unique to each woman. Begin by tuning into your desires. This can be as simple as exploring what makes you feel good and what doesn't. Sometimes, journaling about your thoughts and experiences can provide clarity. It might even help to create a list of what you're curious to try or what's most enjoyable for you.

The process of setting boundaries is equally vital to empowerment. Clearly defined boundaries not only protect your well-being but also communicate respect for yourself and others. It's okay to say no without guilt, and it's okay to change your mind. By establishing and respecting your own limits, you cultivate a sexual environment that feels safe and consensual, which enhances your confidence and desire.

Personal choice is also about tuning into your body and actually listening to what it's telling you. Our bodies are constantly sending us signals—of discomfort, of pleasure, of neutrality—and they often know what we need before our minds do. Pay attention to your natural rhythms and what makes you feel alive and energised. Whether it's feeling empowered in a piece of lingerie or through movement like dance, acknowledging these sensations can deepen your connection with yourself.

There's undeniable power in education. Arm yourself with knowledge about female desire, sexual health, and the complexities that underpin low libido. The more informed you are, the more strategies you can tailor to suit your needs. Women often find it liberating to understand the scientific aspects of their libido, which then equips them to challenge any existing myths or misconceptions they might unknowingly hold.

Challenging societal norms plays a crucial role in empowering personal choices. For centuries, women's sexuality has been shaped by external perceptions rather than internal truths. Recognising and rejecting these societal pressures opens the door to define your own sexuality on your terms. For many, this may involve redefining what 'normal' looks like for your desire, which can be an empowering act of rebellion against what's often imposed by media or culture.

Empowerment arises from the willingness to experiment and explore new avenues of desire. Be it through trying new activities with a partner, delving into solo exploration, or even engaging with erotica and other forms of sensual literature to discover what ignites your passion. It's about finding what resonates with you personally and how these experiences can transform your understanding of your own libido.

Open communication with partners can significantly bolster empowerment. Far too often, the fear of rejection or embarrassment silences many, limiting their sexual satisfaction and growth. Instead, fostering a dialogue about likes, dislikes, and fantasies enriches your intimate bonds. When you're truthful about your desires, you're advocating for your authentic self, which can fortify relationships and promote a deeper form of intimacy.

Our choices are not made in a vacuum, and therefore reaching out for support is a powerful choice in itself. Whether it's seeking guidance from friends, a therapist, or a support group, connecting with others can offer reassurance and insight, affirming that your journey is shared by many and that it's okay to seek help when needed.

Self-care is an important pillar in empowering personal choices. Taking time to nurture yourself in ways that improve both mental and physical health can have profound effects on libido. This might take the form of a relaxing bath, a mindfulness routine, or simply allowing yourself the grace to rest. Choosing self-care is an affirmation of your worth and can rejuvenate your spirit, making room for desire to naturally flow.

Ultimately, empowering personal choices lies in reclaiming the narrative of your sexual health. Each woman's journey is distinct, marked by her own preferences, challenges, and triumphs. Embrace the quest of discovery with a compass of self-love, and let each empowered step forward bring you closer to a fulfilling, liberated sexual life.

Just remember, empowering your journey is a continual process— a beautiful evolution towards embracing the fullness of who you are as a sexual being. With every informed choice made, every boundary respected, every new experience embraced, you're not only advocating for the life you desire but also paving the way for a more enriched intimate existence.

Chapter 21:
Long-term Strategies for Libido Health

As we venture into the realm of long-term strategies for libido health, setting intentions becomes a cornerstone for maintaining a vibrant sexual life. Intentionality invites us to consciously nourish our desires, fostering a continuous connection with our bodies and partners. It's about creating routines that integrate pleasure and self-care, turning practices into habits that sustain libido over time. Focus on consistent communication, both with yourself and your partner, to understand the evolving nature of your desires. Holistic wellness, encompassing balanced nutrition, regular physical activity, and mindfulness techniques, plays a pivotal role in nurturing sexual vitality. Embrace adaptability and patience, as the journey to sustained sexual wellness isn't a quick fix, but rather a fulfilling path of exploration and growth. By cultivating this proactive approach, you're not just addressing low libido; you're championing a lifelong journey toward enhanced intimacy and a richer, more fulfilling sexual experience.

Setting Intention for Desire

In a world that often demands our attention in a thousand different directions, setting an intention for desire can seem like a radical act of self-care. It's about carving out a space for your sexuality, recognising it as a vital part of your identity and well-being. So, why is it important to set an intention for desire? Because it shifts your focus from a passive role to an active one, aligning your actions with your desires and creating a pathway towards a more fulfilling sexual life.

At its core, setting an intention is about clarity and direction. In terms of libido health, it requires an understanding of your personal desire landscape—how you define desire, what stimulates it, and what might be holding it back. Many women find that their libido ebbs and flows, influenced by numerous factors like stress, hormonal changes, and relationship dynamics. By setting a clear intention, you're acknowledging these influences without letting them dictate your desires completely.

Begin by reflecting on what sparks your desire. Consider journaling about the times you felt your libido was at its peak. What circumstances surrounded these moments? Was it a feeling of confidence, an emotional connection with a partner, or a lack of stress? These reflections can serve as a guide, helping you recognise patterns and scenarios that positively influence your libido.

Creating rituals can be a powerful way to reinforce your intentions. Rituals are more than just routine; they hold a deeper meaning, anchoring your intention in everyday life. Whether it's lighting a candle, indulging in a soothing bath, or practicing self-reflection, these personal rituals serve as a reminder of your commitment to nurturing your desire. They distinguish regular activities from those that hold sensual significance.

Another crucial aspect of setting intention is communication, both with yourself and with your partner. Clearly expressing your sexual wants and needs can sometimes be intimidating, but it's an essential step. It involves being honest and open about what you desire, and just as importantly, what you don't. This transparency not only strengthens your relationship but also reinforces your own intention to prioritise your libido health.

Furthermore, it's important to remain flexible in your intentions. Life is inherently unpredictable, and what works for you in one phase might not in another. Adjusting your intentions as you grow and as circumstances change ensures that they remain relevant and empowering. This adaptability prevents frustration and burnout, keeping your journey towards libido health positive and progressive.

Mindfulness practices play a significant role in setting intention. They encourage you to remain present, fostering an awareness that helps quiet the incessant chatter of the mind. Techniques like mindful breathing or meditation can create mental space, enabling you to focus on your body's sensations and signals without judgement. This attentiveness fosters a deeper connection with your sexual self.

Remember, setting an intention is deeply personal; there's no right or wrong way to do it. The act itself is an expression of self-love and empowerment. It's about honouring your sexual desire and giving it the attention it deserves. This positive affirmation helps dismantle any internalised shame or guilt, replacing it with a sense of ownership and pride in your sexual health journey.

Finally, don't underestimate the power of self-compassion in this process. Embracing your libido, with all its complexities and fluctuations, requires patience and kindness towards yourself. Celebrate your progress, however small, and view any setbacks not as failures but as learning experiences. Every step you take towards understanding and enhancing your desire is a stride towards a healthier, more satisfying sexual life.

As you venture into setting intentions for your desire, envision how it'd feel to live in alignment with these intentions. Picture the joy, satisfaction, and connection that a fuller, more vibrant libido might bring to your life and relationships. This vision is not a distant dream but a tangible goal, achievable through the thoughtful setting and nurturing of intention.

Maintaining Sexual Wellness

In the journey to rediscovering your libido, maintaining sexual wellness is not just about quick fixes but creating sustainable, long-term practices. By understanding the importance of ongoing care and attention, you can nurture your sexual health in ways that are both fulfilling and meaningful. Let's explore how you can develop a lifestyle that supports and maintains sexual wellness over the long haul.

Maintaining sexual wellness starts with a deep commitment to self-care. This isn't just about taking bubble baths or indulging in the occasional massage; it's about recognising your unique needs and consistently putting them at the forefront. Prioritise sleep, as rest is fundamental to both mental and physical health, impacting everything from hormone balance to mood. When you're well-rested, your body is better equipped to function optimally, potentially heightening both physical sensations and emotional receptivity.

Nutrition plays a crucial role in maintaining sexual wellness. A diet rich in vitamins, minerals, and essential nutrients supports overall health, including your libido. Foods high in Omega-3 fatty acids, such as salmon and flaxseeds, can enhance circulation, which is crucial for sexual arousal. Similarly, incorporating a variety of fruits, vegetables, lean proteins, and whole grains can boost your energy levels and hormone production. Mindfully choosing what you eat is a form of self-respect, acknowledging the important connection between your diet and your desire.

Exercise is not to be overlooked. Regular physical activity can not only improve your cardiovascular health and boost your energy, but it can also elevate mood by releasing endorphins, the body's natural feel-good hormones. Exercise also promotes a positive body image, which is often linked to a healthy libido. Find an activity you love—be it yoga, dancing, running, or swimming—and make it a regular part of your routine to keep your body and spirit invigorated.

Beyond the physical aspects, mental and emotional care is vital. Practices such as mindfulness and meditation can help reduce stress levels, which, as we've explored, can significantly impact libido. Engaging in daily mindfulness exercises, even for just a few minutes, can bring greater awareness to your feelings and sensations, enhancing your overall sensual experience. Meditation can help you reconnect with yourself, fostering a deeper understanding of your desires and needs.

Open and honest communication is fundamental to maintaining sexual wellness. Whether it's with a partner, friend, or healthcare professional, sharing your experiences and feelings helps to break down barriers and build support networks. Discuss any concerns or desires with your partner to enhance your emotional connection and intimacy. When you feel heard and understood, a safe space is created for you to explore your sexuality without judgement or fear.

Equally important is the idea of setting boundaries and practising consent. Knowing what you are comfortable with and communicating this clearly can empower you both inside and outside the bedroom. Your needs and desires are of utmost importance, and asserting them helps maintain your sense of self-worth and autonomy in intimate situations. This, in turn, can lead to a more satisfying and fulfilling sexual life.

Regular check-ins with healthcare professionals are also an integral part of maintaining sexual wellness. These consultations can ensure that you are in good health and address any issues related to sexual function. Don't shy away from asking questions about anything that concerns you, whether it's changes in your libido, hormone levels, or the side effects of medications. A proactive approach to your health can not only catch potential problems early but also provide reassurance and peace of mind.

Finally, maintaining sexual wellness involves embracing change and remaining adaptable. As our lives evolve, so do our bodies and desires. Approaching these changes with curiosity rather than fear can be liberating. Consider each phase of life as an opportunity to learn more about yourself and discover new aspects of your sexuality.

In conclusion, sexual wellness is a continuous journey. By fostering a lifestyle that prioritises self-care, balanced nutrition, regular exercise, mental well-being, and open communication, you create the foundation for lasting sexual health. With patience and perseverance, and by embracing change, you'll find that maintaining sexual wellness is not just about keeping desire alive but making it flourish over time.

Conclusion

Culminating this journey, we embrace a deeper understanding of female libido, one that recognises its multi-faceted nature. This book has navigated the intricacies of desire with the nuances and depth they warrant, while offering insights and strategies for those who have felt the weight of low libido. By acknowledging the physical, emotional, and social factors that influence sexual appetite, we offer a path towards rekindling passion and intimacy.

It is essential to remember that you are not alone in this pursuit of sexual wellness. Women from every walk of life encounter moments when their desires wane and confidence falters. Together, we've sifted through scientific explanations and societal expectations, dismantling myths that impose limitations and unveil opportunities for empowerment. Armed with knowledge, women can harness this understanding to navigate their own sexuality with grace and curiosity.

Throughout the pages, there's been an emphasis on self-awareness. Recognising how psychological and physiological choices impact your libido can empower you to make informed decisions. Stress, anxiety, medication—all these elements play a part, yet they don't have to be obstacles. Instead, by understanding how they intertwine with sexual desire, we equip ourselves to confront them head-on.

Relationships often find themselves at the crossroads of love and libido. As communication opens up, so do avenues for deeper connection. This book emphasises the beauty of vulnerability and transparency in intimate relationships, urging partners to engage in honest dialogue about needs and desires. By fostering this communication, you strengthen the bond that forms the foundation of sexual health.

Exploration of self and body should be seen through the lens of celebration rather than critique. Encouraging a more loving perspective on the changes our bodies experience, we've uncovered how confidence can flourish when we relinquish unrealistic standards. When you embrace your unique sensuality, you create a fertile ground for desire to thrive.

The harmony between mind and body serves as the cornerstone of sexual wellness. We've ventured into the world of mindfulness to illustrate how presence can elevate intimacy and deepen mutual understanding. This melding of inner tranquility with sensual exploration unlocks new dimensions of pleasure that many have yet to experience.

Even as technology and modern medicine evolve, they provide both challenges and novel means of engaging with our libido. From holistic therapies to conventional interventions, exploring these avenues offers hope for solutions tailored to individual needs. Embracing these options encourages an open-minded approach to enhancing sexual health.

Ultimately, the call to action is simple—take hold of your sexual health as an integral aspect of your overall well-being. By owning your narrative and advocating for yourself, you wield the power to define what libido and desire mean to you. Passion doesn't have to be stationary or static; it can adapt, shift, and flourish alongside you.

This book has aimed to be a voyage of discovery, a toolkit for transformation. It invites you to keep the conversation about sexuality alive, both within your inner dialogues and your external relationships. Embrace this journey with compassion and persistence, and revel in the intimacy and desire that await. May this newfound knowledge serve as a light, guiding you towards a fulfilled and vibrant sexual life.

In conclusion, the tapestry of eluding desire becomes more vivid and less elusive when painted with understanding, acceptance, and love. The pursuit of a healthy libido isn't a single destination but an ongoing adventure, one that promises continuous growth and evolution. With each chapter closed, a new one unfolds—challenging, inviting, and rewarding. Seize it with courage, as you continue along this evocative path towards sustained sexual wellness.

Appendix A:
Additional Resources

Embarking on a journey to understand and enhance your libido isn't something you have to do alone. There are numerous resources available to support, inspire, and guide you along the way. Start by exploring organisations dedicated to women's sexual health, providing expert advice, counselling, and community support. Many reputable online platforms offer accessible articles and forums where you can connect with others who share similar experiences. Books by leading experts can provide deeper insights and practical strategies, while podcasts and webinars offer engaging, real-time discussions from the comfort of your home. Additionally, consider speaking to healthcare professionals who can tailor advice specifically to your needs, ensuring a comprehensive approach to your sexual wellness. Remember, reaching out for support and seeking knowledge is a powerful step towards reclaiming and celebrating your sexual health and desire.

Support Organisations and Contacts

Finding the right support is crucial on your journey to understanding and enhancing your libido. There are numerous organisations dedicated to providing resources, guidance, and a sense of community. It's important to remember that you're not alone in this process, and these organisations can be valuable allies.

Relate is one of the prominent organisations offering counselling services specifically aimed at individuals and couples experiencing difficulties in their sexual relationships. With a focus on improving communication and understanding within relationships, Relate provides sessions both online and in person. Their services are tailored to help individuals and couples navigate the complexities of sexual desire and build stronger connections.

For women specifically, Women's Health Concern offers informational resources and support for a variety of issues, including sexual health. They provide clear, reliable information and connect women with medical experts who understand the nuanced nature of female libido. One phone call or email can open the door to the support and advice you need.

Additionally, Mind, a leading mental health charity, recognises the profound impact that mental well-being can have on sexual desire. They offer mental health support and services that could help you address issues like anxiety, depression, or stress, which might be affecting your libido. Their free resources and workshops can be a source of comfort and empowerment as you work towards rediscovering your desire.

Furthermore, the Sexual Advice Association provides an invaluable resource for individuals seeking advice on sexual matters, including low libido. They focus on educating the public and healthcare professionals about sexual function and dysfunction, offering a public helpline and informative leaflets. Their website is full of resources that could help you feel more informed and less isolated as you navigate your libido journey.

It's also worth exploring forums and online communities where people share personal experiences and solutions for overcoming low libido. The conversations in these spaces often provide real-world advice and encouragement. Websites like Mumsnet have forums dedicated to discussions about sexual health and well-being, offering peer support from those who have faced similar challenges.

Moreover, if you prefer to seek help through alternative therapies, the College of Sexual and Relationship Therapists (COSRT) lists certified therapists who specialise in a variety of approaches across the UK. Whether you're curious about trying sex therapy or another holistic approach, COSRT can connect you with professionals who have the expertise to guide you on this personal journey.

For those who want immediate access to information about sexual health without contacting organisations directly, books and online articles from authors who specialise in female sexuality can be a worthwhile investment. Reading personal stories and scientific insights can empower you with knowledge and give you new perspectives on your own experiences.

Don't underestimate the power of local community health centres and GP surgeries, which often provide sexual health services and referrals to specialists. These can be great starting points if you prefer more personal, face-to-face discussions about your sexual health needs and concerns.

Also consider contacting your national NHS service. They've continually expanded their resources and educational materials regarding sexual health, ensuring that their offerings include guidance specific to female libido. The NHS website features reliable, evidence-based information and links to local services, which can be reassuring when you're seeking quality advice.

Finally, if you're in a situation where immediate support is necessary, the Samaritans offer a helpline where you can speak with someone who will listen without judgement, 24/7. Although not specific to sexual health, their empathetic listeners can provide emotional support and may suggest ways to access further help.

Creating a support network through these organisations can be transformative, giving you the tools and connections needed to work through any difficulties related to low libido. By reaching out, you're taking a powerful step towards a more fulfilling and empowered sexual life.

www.ingramcontent.com/pod-product-compliance
Lightning Source LLC
Chambersburg PA
CBHW020437290526
45785CB00002B/888